BASIC GUIDE TO
MEDICAL EMERGENCIES
IN THE DENTAL PRACTICE

BASIC GUIDE TO MEDICAL EMERGENCIES IN THE DENTAL PRACTICE

Phil Jevon

RN, BSc(Hons), PGCE, ENB 124

Resuscitation Officer/Clinical Skills Lead
Honorary Clinical Lecturer
Walsall Hospital
Walsall
UK

Consulting Editors

Celia Strickland, BDS Dental Practitioner, Staffordshire, UK

Tessa Meese, RDN, Cert OHE, LCGi, DCP Tutor, Postgraduate Office, NHS West Midlands, St Chad's Court, Birmingham, UK

Jagtar Singh Pooni, BSc(Hons), MRCP (England), FRCA, Consultant in Anaesthesia & Intensive Care Medicine, New Cross Hospital, Wolverhampton, UK

WILEY-BLACKWELL
A John Wiley & Sons, Ltd., Publication

This edition first published 2010
© 2010 Phil Jevon

Blackwell Publishing was acquired by John Wiley & Sons in February 2007.
Blackwell's publishing programme has been merged with Wiley's global Scientific, Technical,
and Medical business to form Wiley-Blackwell.

Registered office
John Wiley & Sons Ltd, The Atrium, Southern Gate, Chichester, West Sussex, PO19 8SQ,
United Kingdom

Editorial offices
9600 Garsington Road, Oxford, OX4 2DQ, United Kingdom
2121 State Avenue, Ames, Iowa 50014-8300, USA

For details of our global editorial offices, for customer services and for information about how to
apply for permission to reuse the copyright material in this book please see our website at
www.wiley.com/wiley-blackwell.

The right of the author to be identified as the author of this work has been asserted in accordance
with the Copyright, Designs and Patents Act 1988.

Library of Congress Cataloging-in-Publication Data
Jevon, Philip.
Basic guide to medical emergencies in the dental practice / Phil Jevon ; consulting editors,
Celia Strickland, Tessa Meese, Jagtar Singh Pooni.
p. ; cm. – (Basic guide to dentistry series)
Includes bibliographical references and index.
ISBN 978-1-4051-9784-7 (pbk. : alk. paper) 1. Dentistry. 2. Medical emergencies. 3. Dental
emergencies. I. Title. II. Series: Basic guide to dentistry series.
[DNLM: 1. Emergency Treatment–methods. 2. Dental Care–methods. 3. Emergencies.
WU 105 J58b 2010]
RK51.5.J475 2010
617.6'026–dc22
2009033616

A catalogue record for this book is available from the British Library.

Set in 10/12.5 pt Sabon by Aptara® Inc., New Delhi, India
Printed and bound in Malaysia by KHL Printing Co Sdn Bhd

1   2010

Contents

Foreword

We all hope that a serious medical emergency will not happen in our practice, but at some stage it probably will. I was just 20 years old and a dental student when I witnessed someone no older than me having a cardiac arrest. This young man had been involved in a major accident and was on a hospital ward at the time. There was a crash team on hand and many skilled people to play a part in the team who tried to save him. At that moment I learnt that I was now a dental professional and I needed to know what to do in the case of any medical emergency. It happens and we need to be prepared. That young man died that day. Things do not always turn out well but we can do everything in our power to help make sure there is the best chance possible.

Whatever our role is in the dental team we can play our part. This view will help us know what to do and when to do it. This may be in the dental surgery, the waiting room, the office, or at other times in our lives. Patients and the public more widely rely on us to protect their safety.

This book provides you with an evidence based approach which follows national guidelines. The text gives a systematic approach to care and images describing the procedures will help you follow them. The book provides information about automated external defibrillation which is a new concept in the dental practice.

This book will be useful to all members of the dental team and especially helpful for dentists, dental therapists and hygienists and dental nurses.

Karen Elley
Postgraduate Dental Dean
BDS, FDS RCS, DDPH RCS, MCDH, FFPH, Cert Med Ed
West Midlands

Acknowledgements

I am grateful to the following:

Celia Strickland, Tessa Meese and Jag Pooni for their helpful suggestions to improve the book.

Karen Elley for writing the Foreword.

Richard Griffith for writing the legal chapter.

Shareen Juwle, Steve Webb, Stuart Hildage and the dental nurses at the Manor Hospital Walsall for their help with the photographs.

The staff at Wiley-Blackwell for their help and support.

Katrina Hulme-Cross for commissioning the book!

Chapter 1

Medical emergencies and resuscitation in the dental practice: an overview

INTRODUCTION

Dental practitioners have a duty of care to ensure that an effective and safe service is provided for their patients. The satisfactory performance in a medical emergency or in a resuscitation attempt in the dental practice has wide-ranging implications in terms of resuscitation equipment, resuscitation training, standards of care, clinical governance, risk management and clinical audit (Jevon, 2002). The Resuscitation Council (UK) (2006) has issued standards for clinical practice and training in medical emergencies and resuscitation for dental practitioners and dental care professionals in general dental practice.

The aim of this chapter is to provide an overview of the management of medical emergencies and resuscitation in the dental practice.

LEARNING OUTCOMES

At the end of the chapter the reader will be able to:

- Discuss the concept of the chain of survival

- Discuss the incidence of medical emergencies in the dental practice

- Outline the General Dental Council guidelines on medical emergencies

- Summarise the Resuscitation Council UK statement: *Medical emergencies and resuscitation standards for clinical practice and training for dental practitioners and dental care professionals in general dental practice*

- Discuss the principles of safer handling during cardiopulmonary resuscitation

- Outline the procedure for calling 999 for an ambulance

CONCEPT OF THE CHAIN OF SURVIVAL

Survival from cardiac arrest relies on a sequence of time-sensitive interventions (Nolan *et al.*, 2006). The concept of the original chain of survival emphasised that each time-sensitive intervention must be optimised in order to maximise the chance of survival: a chain is only as strong as its weakest link (Cummins *et al.*, 1991).

The chain of survival was revised in 2005 (Figure 1.1) to stress the importance of recognising critical illness and/or angina and preventing cardiac arrest (both in and out of hospital) and post-resuscitation care (Nolan, 2005):

- *Early recognition and call for help to prevent cardiac arrest:* this link stresses the importance of recognising patients at risk of cardiac arrest, dialing 999 for the emergency services and providing effective treatment to hopefully prevent cardiac arrest (Nolan *et al.*, 2006); most patients sustaining an out-of-hospital cardiac arrest display warning symptoms for a significant duration before the event (Müller *et al.*, 2006).

- *Early CPR to buy time* and *Early defibrillation to restart the heart:* the two central links in the chain stress the importance of linking CPR and

Figure 1.1 Chain of survival. Reproduced with permission from Laerdal Medical Ltd, Orpington, Kent, UK.

defibrillation as essential components of early resuscitation in an attempt to restore life.

- *Post-resuscitation care to restore quality of life:* the priority is to preserve cerebral and myocardial function and to restore quality of life (Nolan *et al.*, 2006).

INCIDENCE OF MEDICAL EMERGENCIES IN DENTAL PRACTICE

The incidence of medical emergencies in dental practice is very low. Medical emergencies occur in hospital dental practice more frequently, but in similar proportions to that found in general dental practice (Atherton *et al.*, 2000). With the elderly population in dental practices increasing, medical emergencies in the dental practice will undoubtedly occur (Dym, 2008).

A literature search for published surveys on the incidence of medical emergencies and resuscitation in the dental practice found the following,

Survey of dental practitioners in Australia

A postal questionnaire survey of 1250 general dental practitioners undertaken in Australia (Chapman, 1997) found that:

- one in seven (14%) had had to resuscitate a patient;
- the most common medical emergencies encountered were adverse reactions to local anaesthetics, grand mal seizures, angina and hypoglycaemia.

Survey of dentists in England

A survey of dentists (Girdler & Smith, 1999) (300 responded) in England found that over a 12-month period they had encountered:

- vasovagal syncope (63%) – 596 patients affected;
- angina (12%) – 53 patients affected;
- hypoglycaemia (10%) – 54 patients affected;
- epileptic fit (10%) – 42 patients affected;
- choking (5%) – 27 patients affected;
- asthma (5%) – 20 patients affected;
- cardiac arrest (0.3%) – 1 patient affected.

Survey of dental practitioners in a UK university dental hospital

Atherton *et al.* (2000) assessed the frequency of medical emergencies by undertaking a survey of clinical staff (dentists, hygienists, nurses and radiographers) at a university dental hospital. The researchers found that:

- fainting was the commonest event;
- other medical emergency events were experienced with an average frequency of 1.8 events per year;
- highest frequency of emergencies were reported by staff in oral surgery.

Survey of dentists in New Zealand

A total of 199 dentists responded to a postal survey undertaken by Broadbent and Thomson (2001) in New Zealand, with the following findings:

- Medical emergencies had occurred in 129 practices (65.2%) within the previous 10 years (mean – 2.0 events per 10,000 patients treated under local analgesia, other forms of pain control, or sedation);
- Vasovagal events were the most common emergencies occurring in 121 (61.1%) practices within the previous year (mean 6.9 events per 10,000 patients treated under local analgesia, other forms of pain control, or sedation).

Survey of dental staff in Ohio

A survey of dental staff in Ohio (Kandray *et al.*, 2007) found that 5% had performed CPR on a patient in their dental surgery.

Survey of dentists in Germany

A survey of 620 dentists in Germany (Müller *et al.*, 2008) found that in a 12-month period:

- 57% had encountered up to 3 emergencies;
- 36% had encountered up to 10 emergencies;
- Vasovagal episode was the most common reported emergency – average 2 per dentist;
- 42 dentists (7%) had encountered an epileptic fit;

- 24 dentists (4%) had encountered an asthma attack;

- 5 dentists (0.8%) had encountered choking;

- 7 dentists (1.1%) had encountered anaphylaxis;

- 2 dentists (0.3%) had encountered a cardiopulmonary arrest.

GENERAL DENTAL COUNCIL GUIDELINES ON MEDICAL EMERGENCIES

Standards for Dental Professionals (General Dental Council, 2005) emphasises that all dental professionals are responsible for putting patients' interests first, and acting to protect them. Central to this responsibility is the need for dental professionals to ensure that they are able to deal with medical emergencies that may arise in their practice. Such emergencies are, fortunately, a rare occurrence, but it is important to recognise that a medical emergency could happen at any time and that all members of the dental team need to know their role in the event of one occurring.

The General Dental Council, in its publication *Principles of Dental Team Working* (GDC, 2006), states that the person who employs, manages or leads a team in a dental practice should ensure that:

- There are arrangements for at least two people available to deal with medical emergencies when treatment is planned to take place;

- All members of staff, not just the registered team members, know their role if a patient collapses or there is another kind of medical emergency;

- All members of staff who might be involved in dealing with a medical emergency are trained and prepared to deal with such an emergency at any time;

- Members of the team practise together regularly in a simulated emergency so they know exactly what to do.

Maintaining the knowledge and competence to deal with medical emergencies is an important aspect of all dental professionals' continuing professional development (GDC, 2006). The above guidance has been endorsed in the Resuscitation Council (UK) statement.

RESUSCITATION COUNCIL (UK) STATEMENT

The Resuscitation Council (UK)'s statement *Medical emergencies and resuscitation standards for clinical practice and training for dental practitioners and dental care professionals in general dental practice* (2006) provides guidance and recommendations concerning medical emergencies that may occur in the dental practice. It was revised in 2008 to incorporate the new anaphylaxis guidelines. It has been endorsed by the General Dental Council.

Contributors

Contributors to this statement included:

- members of the Resuscitation Council (UK);
- a consultant in oral medicine;
- dental practitioners;
- chairman of the British Dental Association Formulary Committee;
- chairman of the British Dental Association Practice Managers and Service Committee;
- president-elect of the Society for Advancement of Anaesthesia in Dentistry;
- an Executive Committee Member of the Dental Sedation Teachers Group.

Topics covered

Topics covered include medical risk assessment, resuscitation procedures and equipment, and the use of emergency drugs in general dental practice. It also includes topics such as staff training, patient transfer and post-resuscitation/emergency care.

Key recommendations

The key recommendations in the statement are that:

- Every dental practice should have a procedure in place for medical risk assessment of their patients;
- All Dental Practitioners and Dental Care Professionals should follow the systematic 'ABCDE' approach when assessing an acutely sick patient;
- Specific emergency drugs and items of emergency medical equipment should be immediately available in every dental practice (this should be standardised throughout the UK);

- Every clinical area should have immediate access to an automated external defibrillator (AED);

- Dental practitioners and dental care professionals should receive training in cardiopulmonary resuscitation (CPR), including basic airway management and the use of an AED, with annual updates;

- Regular simulated emergency scenarios should take place in the dental practice;

- Dental practices should have a protocol in place for calling medical assistance in an emergency (this will usually be calling 999 for an ambulance);

- All medical emergencies should be audited.

Further information

For further information, access the Resuscitation Council (UK)'s website (http://www.resus.org.uk/pages/MEdental.pdf).

ABCDE ASSESSMENT OF THE SICK PATIENT

Many people who suffer an out-of-hospital cardiac arrest display warning symptoms for a significant duration before collapse (Müller *et al.*, 2006). These symptoms could include:

- chest pain;

- dyspnoea (breathlessness);

- nausea/vomiting;

- dizziness/syncope.
  (Müller *et al.*, 2006).

The Resuscitation Council (UK) (2006) recommends the ABCDE approach to assess the sick patient (see chapter 3). All dental professionals should be familiar with the approach because, not only will it help them to recognise the warning symptoms which many people exhibit prior to sudden cardiac arrest, but also it will help to establish whether the patient is sick or not.

The logical and systematic ABCDE approach to assessing the sick patient incorporates:

- airway;

- breathing;

- circulation;
- disability;
- exposure.

When assessing the patient, a complete initial assessment should be undertaken, identifying and treating life-threatening problems first, before moving on to the next part of assessment. The effectiveness of treatment/intervention should be evaluated, and regular reassessment undertaken. The need to call for an ambulance should be recognised and other members of the multidisciplinary team should be utilised as appropriate so that patient assessment, instigation of appropriate monitoring and interventions can be undertaken.

MEDICAL RISK ASSESSMENT IN GENERAL DENTAL PRACTICE

Although any patient could experience a medical emergency in general practice, certain patients will be at great higher risk. It is therefore important to identify these patients by undertaking medical and medication histories. The dental practitioner can then take measures to reduce the chance of a problem arising in dental practice.

History taking

Medical and medication histories should be obtained by the dental practitioner and should not be delegated to another member of the dental team; if a patient completes a health questionnaire it is only acceptable if augmented by a verbal history taken by the dental practitioner (Resuscitation Council (UK), 2006). For some patients, it may be necessary to modify the planned treatment or even refer them for treatment in hospital.

Risk stratification scoring system

A risk stratification scoring system, e.g. the American Society of Anaesthesiologists' classification, should be used routinely by the dental practitioner when assessing a patient for dental treatment, as it may help to identify those patients who are at greater risk of a medical emergency during dental treatment (Resuscitation Council (UK), 2006). It should trigger hospital referral for treatment if a certain level of risk is attained. It has been suggested that a risk stratification could be incorporated into the routine medical history questionnaire so that all patients are risk assessed (Resuscitation Council (UK), 2006).

Up-to-date patient details

It is recommended to update the patient's medical and medication histories on a regular basis (at least annually) or more frequently as required; it may be necessary to liaise with the patient's general practitioner (Resuscitation Council (UK), 2006).

Existing medical problem

Patients with certain existing medical problems are more likely to suffer a medical emergency in the dental surgery:

- *Angina:* if a patient has frequent episodes of angina following exertion or suffers from angina which is easily provoked, he or she may experience an episode of angina in the dental practice. If the patient suffers from angina episodes caused by anxiety or stress, he may benefit from being prescribed an oral anxiolytic drug, e.g. diazepam, before dental treatment. *Note:* prolonged drug treatment may lead to dependence (British Medical Association & the Royal Pharmaceutical Society (2008). The patient should be considered at higher risk if he or she has unstable angina, angina episodes at night or has had a recent admission to hospital with angina. For these patients, in-hospital treatment may be prudent (Resuscitation Council (UK), 2006).

- *Asthma:* an asthmatic patient is more likely to have a severe asthma attack in the dental practice if he or she has had a previous near-fatal asthmatic episode, if he has been admitted to the emergency department with asthma in the previous 12 months, or if he has been prescribed three or more classes of medication, or if he regularly requires beta-2 agonist therapy (British Thoracic Society, 2008).

- *Epilepsy:* the patient will usually be able to provide the dental practitioner with a good indication of how well his condition is controlled. There is a greater risk of having a fit in the dental practice if his fits are poorly controlled or if his medications have recently been altered. It would be prudent to ascertain the timing of, and precipitating factors for, the patient's last three fits (Resuscitation Council UK, 2006).

- *Diabetes:* a patient with type 1 diabetes (on insulin) is more likely become hypoglycaemic in the dental practice than a patient with type 2 diabetes (diet or tablet controlled); patients whose diabetes is poorly controlled or who have poor awareness of their hypoglycaemic episodes are more likely to develop hypoglycaemia (Resuscitation Council (UK), 2006).

- *Allergies:* it is important to ascertain whether the patient has any known allergies, particularly to local anaesthetic, antibiotics or latex. If the patient has a severe latex allergy, use latex-free gloves; if the patient has a severe latex allergy, he should either be treated in a hospital environment or in a latex-free dental environment where appropriate resuscitation facilities are at hand (Resuscitation Council (UK), 2006).

PRINCIPLES OF SAFER HANDLING DURING CARDIOPULMONARY RESUSCITATION

The Resuscitation Council (UK), in its publication *Guidance for Safer Handling during Resuscitation in Hospitals* (2001), has issued guidelines concerning safer handling during cardiopulmonary resuscitation. Although specifically aimed at hospital staff, the guidelines can be adapted for use when performing cardiopulmonary resuscitation in the dental practice. An overview will now be provided. Although the use of slide sheets is recommended when moving the patient, these are not usually available in the dental practice.

Cardiac arrest on the floor

- If the patient has collapsed on the floor, e.g. in the waiting room, perform cardiopulmonary resuscitation on the floor. If the area has restricted access, consider sliding the patient across the floor.

- Ventilation: kneel behind the patient's head ensuring the knees are shoulder-width apart, rest back to sit on the heels and lean forwards from the hips towards the patient's face.

- Chest compressions: kneel at the side of the patient, level with his chest, and adopt a high kneeling position with the knees shoulder-width apart; position the shoulders directly over the patient's sternum and keeping the arms straight compress the chest ensuring the force for compressions results from flexing the hips.

Cardiac arrest in the dental chair

- Remove any environmental hazards, e.g. mouthwash, dental instrument tray.

- Lower the chair into a horizontal position.

- Ventilation: to use the mask device, ideally sit on the dentist's stool at the head end of the chair. The person squeezing the bag should stand with their feet in a walk/stand position facing the patient; avoid prolonged static postures.

- Chest compressions: ensure the chair is at a height which places the patient between the knee and mid-thigh of the person performing chest compressions; stand at the side of the chair with the feet shoulder-width apart, position the shoulders directly over the patient's sternum and, keeping the arms straight, compress the chest, ensuring the force for compressions results from flexing the hips.

Cardiac arrest in a chair in the waiting room

- Lowering the patient to the floor: with two colleagues, slide the patient on to the floor; one should support the patient's head during the procedure.

Cardiac arrest in the toilet

- Ensure the toilet door is kept open and access maintained.

- Lowering the patient to the floor: with two colleagues, slide the patient on to the floor; one should support the patient's head during the procedure.

PROCEDURE FOR CALLING 999 FOR AN AMBULANCE

There are many emergency situations in the dental practice which will require an ambulance to be called, e.g. chest pain, difficulty with breathing, anaphylaxis and cardiopulmonary arrest. When calling 999 for an ambulance, the following is a suggested procedure.

- If available, obtain the 'when dialing 999 information card' which will have the dental practice's address, telephone number and any specific instructions or guidelines if the practice is difficult to find. Reading from this card will make it easier for the person calling 999 for an ambulance and will help minimise the risk of incorrect information being given.

- Lift the telephone receiver or switch the phone on and dial 999 (when using a telephone in a dental practice it is usually necessary to access an outside line first, e.g. by pressing a specific key or pressing 9).

- When the telephone operator answers, he or she will ask which emergency service you require. Tell the operator that you need an ambulance and you will then be connected to the ambulance service. (It is important to remember that 999 (or 112) is used for other emergencies as well such as the fire service, police, mountain rescue, coastguard.)

- Once connected to the ambulance service, the ambulance control officer (Figure 1.2) will ask you where you would like the ambulance to come to, the telephone number of the phone you are calling from and details of the emergency. Give accurate details of the address or location where help is needed. If there is a recognisable landmark, e.g. famous shop nearby, this information will be helpful. An ambulance or paramedic on a motorcycle will be dispatched (Figure 1.3a,b).

Figure 1.2 Ambulance control centre. Reproduced with kind permission from West Midlands Ambulance Service.

(a)   (b)

Figure 1.3 (a) Ambulance. Reproduced with kind permission from West Midlands Ambulance Service. (b) Paramedic on a motorcycle. Reproduced with kind permission from West Midlands Ambulance Service.

- If appropriate, stay on the line and continue to listen to important advice provided by the ambulance control officer.

- Confirm with the senior dental practitioner that an ambulance has been called.

- Note the time the 999 call was made.

- If possible, ask someone to wait outside the dental practice to attract the attention of the ambulance when it draws near (a patient may be willing to do this).

It is important to:

- stay calm;

- listen carefully to any questions the operator may ask;

- speak slowly and clearly; do not shout.

CONCLUSION

Dental practitioners have a duty of care to ensure that an effective and safe service is provided for their patients. This chapter has provided an overview of the management of medical emergencies and resuscitation with specific reference to the standards for clinical practice and training in medical emergencies and resuscitation for dental practitioners and dental care professionals in general dental practice.

REFERENCES

Atherton G, Pemberton M, Thornhill M (2000) Medical emergencies: the experience of staff of a UK dental teaching hospital. *British Dental Journal*; 12;189(3):123.

British Medical Association & the Royal Pharmaceutical Society of Great Britain (2008) *British National Formulary 56*. Royal Pharmaceutical Society, London.

British Thoracic Society (2008) *2008 British Guideline on the Management of Asthma*. British Thoracic Society, London.

Broadbent J, Thomson W (2001) The readiness of New Zealand general dental practitioners for medical emergencies. *New Zealand Dental Journal*; 97(429):82–86.

Chapman P (1997) Medical emergencies in dental practice and choice of emergency drugs and equipment: a survey of Australian dentists. *Australian Dental Journal*; 42(2):103–108.

Cummins R, Ornato J, Thies W, Pepe P (1991) Improving survival from sudden cardiac arrest: the "chain of survival" concept. A statement for health professionals from the Advanced Cardiac Life Support Subcommittee and the Emergency Cardiac Care Committee, American Heart Association. *Circulation*; 83:1832–1847.

Dym H (2008) Preparing the dental office for medical emergencies. *Dental Clinics of North America*; 52(3):605–608.

General Dental Council (2005) *Standards for Dental Professionals*. GDC, London.

General Dental Council (2006) *Principles of Dental Team Working*. GDC, London.

Girdler N, Smith D (1999) Prevalence of emergency events in British dental practice and emergency management skills of British dentists. *Resuscitation*; 41:159–167.

Jevon P (2002) *Advanced Cardiac Life Support*. Butterworth Heinemann, Oxford.

Kandray D, Pieren J, Benner R (2007) Attitudes of Ohio dentists and dental hygienists on the use of automated external defibrillators. *Journal of Dental Education*; 71(4):480–486.

Müller D, Agrawal R, Arntz H (2006) How sudden is sudden cardiac death? *Circulation*; 114:1146–1150.

Müller M, Hänsel M, Stehr S *et al.* (2008) A state-wide survey of medical emergency management in dental practices: incidence of emergencies and training experience *Emergency Medicine Journal*; 25;296–300.

Nolan J (2005) European Resuscitation Council Guidelines for Resuscitation 2005. Section 1: Introduction. *Resuscitation*; 67(Suppl. 1):S3–6.

Nolan J, Soar J, Eikeland H (2006) Image in resuscitation: the chain of survival. *Resuscitation*; 71:270–271.

Resuscitation Council UK (2001) *Guidance for Safer Handling during Resuscitation in Hospitals*. Resuscitation Council (UK), London.

Resuscitation Council UK (2006) *Medical emergencies and resuscitation standards for clinical practice and training for dental practitioners and dental care professionals in general dental practice*. Resuscitation Council (UK), London.

Chapter 2

Resuscitation equipment in the dental practice

INTRODUCTION

Successful resuscitation partly relies on the availability and correct functioning of resuscitation equipment (Dyson & Smith, 2002). The Resuscitation Council (UK) (2006) has made recommendations on the provision and use of resuscitation equipment in the dental practice. Other additional equipment will be required if the dental practice undertakes sedation.

All dental staff who may be involved in dealing with a cardiopulmonary arrest or a medical emergency must be prepared to deal with it (General Dental Council, 2006). Procedures must therefore be in place to ensure that the recommended resuscitation equipment is immediately available and in working order. In addition, dental staff must know where it is stored within their working area and how to use it safely and effectively (Resuscitation Council UK, 2006).

The aim of this chapter is to discuss the provision of resuscitation equipment in the dental practice.

LEARNING OUTCOMES

At the end of this chapter the reader will be able to:

- List the recommended minimum resuscitation equipment in the dental practice
- Discuss the routine checking of emergency equipment
- Discuss the checking of emergency equipment following use

RECOMMENDED MINIMUM RESUSCITATION EQUIPMENT IN THE DENTAL PRACTICE

The Resuscitation Council (UK) (2006) recommends the following minimum equipment for the management of a medical emergency or cardiopulmonary arrest in the dental practice.

Airway equipment

- Set of oropharyngeal airways sizes 1, 2, 3 and 4 (Figure 2.1).

- Portable suction device with appropriate suction catheters and tubing (Figure 2.2), e.g. Yankauer Sucker.

Figure 2.1 Oropharyngeal airways.

Figure 2.2 Portable suction device. Reproduced with kind permission from Timesco, Basildon, UK.

Breathing equipment

- Pocket mask with oxygen port (Figure 2.3).

- Self-inflating resuscitation bag with oxygen reservoir and tubing (Figure 2.4) (if local staff have been trained to use it).

- Selection of well-fitting adult and child face masks for attaching to the self-inflating bag.

- Oxygen face mask with tubing (Figure 2.5).

Figure 2.3 Pocket mask with oxygen port.

Figure 2.4 Self-inflating resuscitation bag with oxygen reservoir and tubing.

Figure 2.5 Oxygen face mask with tubing.

(a)   (b)

Figure 2.6 (a) Portable oxygen cylinder (D size) with (b) pressure reduction valve and flowmeter.

- Portable oxygen cylinder (D size) with pressure reduction valve and flowmeter (Figure 2.6).
- Oxygen cylinder key (if appropriate).
- 'Spacer device' for inhaled bronchodilator.

Circulation equipment

- Automated external defibrillator (AED) (Figure 2.7) (with defibrillation electrodes, pair of heavy duty scissors and a razor).
- Sterile syringes and needles.

(a)

(b)

(c)

(d)

Figure 2.7 Automated external defibrillator (AED) (a) closed, (b) open, with (c) defibrillation electrodes, a pair of heavy-duty scissors and a razor, and (d) adult pads.

Drugs

- Glyceryl trinitrate (GTN) spray (400 μg/dose).

- Salbutamol aerosol inhaler (100 μg/actuation).

- Adrenaline injection (1:1,000, 1 mg/ml).

- Aspirin 300 mg dispersable.

- Glucagon injection 1 mg.

- Oral glucose solution/tablets/gel/powder.

- Midazolam 5 mg/ml or 10 mg/ml (buccal or intranasal).

Additional items

- Automated blood glucose measurement device (Figure 2.8).
- Gloves.

Figure 2.8 Automated blood glucose measurement device.

Resuscitation bag

It would be helpful if the resuscitation equipment was stored in an easily accessible 'grab-bag' or similar. This bag should be spacious, sturdy, easily accessible and portable.

CHECKING RESUSCITATION EQUIPMENT AND DRUGS

The individual dental practice is responsible for checking the resuscitation equipment, the frequency of which will be determined by local circumstances, but should ideally be on a weekly basis (Resuscitation Council (UK), 2006). The responsibility for undertaking the checks should be delegated to a named person(s).

Equipment inventory

Having an equipment inventory is helpful as it will assist the checking of the resuscitation equipment. The regular checks should be recorded and subject to local audit (Resuscitation Council (UK), 2006).

Drugs

Expiry dates of the drugs should be checked and there should be a planned replacement programme in place (Resuscitation Council (UK), 2006).

Figure 2.9 Checking self-inflating resuscitation bag.

Self-inflating bag

The self-inflating bag should be checked to ensure that there are no leaks (Figure 2.9) and that the rim of the face mask is adequately inflated. Older reusable devices should be particularly carefully checked because they are prone to perishing. Ideally, they should be replaced with new single-use (and latex-free) devices.

Defibrillator

If the dental practice has a defibrillator, it should be checked following the manufacturer's recommendations.

Automated external defibrillators

Most AEDs perform self-checks on a daily basis and will alert staff if a problem is identified, e.g. if the battery requires replacement. Generally the only checks required to be undertaken by dental staff are that the device is 'rescue ready' and that the defibrillation electrodes are not out of date.

The 'rescue ready' indicator varies between different makes and models. In the AED depicted in Figure 2.7, a green light indicates that the defibrillator is 'rescue ready'. If the AED is indicating that there is a problem (usually by an audible bleep), this should be investigated and the problem rectified as soon as possible.

Defibrillation electrodes usually have a shelf life of approximately 18 months to two years. Once out of date, they will need to be replaced. A procedure should be in place to ensure that replacement electrodes are ordered in advance.

Most AEDs use lithium batteries that do not require recharging. Once installed in the AED, the battery will last a specified period of time, typically up to 5 years (this will be reduced if the AED is used). There should be a procedure in place to ensure that a new battery is ordered, again in advance of the current one requiring to be replaced.

Some AEDs use a rechargeable battery: it is important to ensure that the battery is charged and recharged following the manufacturer's recommendations. Again, a procedure should be place to ensure that this happens.

Some AEDs need to be kept on charge: it is important to ensure that the AED is kept on charge following the manufacturer's recommendations. Again, a procedure should be place to that ensure this happens.

> Most AEDs do not need to be switched on for checking – doing this will actually run down the battery

Manual defibrillators

Some dental practices have a manual defibrillator. It is usually necessary for this to remain plugged into the mains to ensure that the battery is fully charged in the event of use. It is important to ensure that the appropriate defibrillation gel pads and electrodes are available. It is common practice for manual defibrillators to be maintained and serviced by the electro-biomedical engineers (EBME) department at the local hospital.

Single use and latex free

Ideally, all emergency equipment should be single use and latex free (Resuscitation Council (UK), 2006).

CHECKING RESUSCITATION EQUIPMENT FOLLOWING USE

Checking of resuscitation equipment following use should be a specifically delegated responsibility. As well as the routine checks identified above, any disposable equipment used should be replaced and reusable equipment, e.g. self-inflating bag, cleaned following local infection control procedures and manufacturer's recommendations. Any difficulties with equipment encountered during resuscitation should be documented and reported to relevant personnel.

CONCLUSION

This chapter has detailed what resuscitation equipment should be immediately available in the event of a medical emergency or cardiopulmonary arrest. Suggestions have been made regarding the storage, checking and maintenance of this equipment.

REFERENCES

Dyson E, Smith G (2002) Common faults in resuscitation equipment – guidelines for checking equipment and drugs used in adult cardiopulmonary resuscitation *Resuscitation*; 55(2):137–149.

General Dental Council (2006) *Principles of Dental Team Working.* GDC, London.

Resuscitation Council UK (2006) *Medical emergencies and resuscitation standards for clinical practice and training for dental practitioners and dental care professionals in general dental practice.* Resuscitation Council (UK), London.

Chapter 3

Recognition of the sick patient: the ABCDE approach

INTRODUCTION

The Resuscitation Council (UK) (2006a) recommends the early recognition of the sick patient by undertaking a systematic clinical assessment following the ABCDE approach: pre-empting a medical emergency would allow appropriate help, e.g. ambulance, to be called, hopefully before the patient deteriorates or collapses.

The aim of this chapter is to understand the principles of recognition of the sick patient following the ABCDE approach.

LEARNING OUTCOMES

At the end of this chapter the reader will be able to:

- List the clinical signs of acute illness
- Define the ABCDE approach
- List the general principles of the ABCDE approach
- Describe the ABCDE approach to the sick patient
- Discuss the principles of pulse oximetry
- Describe the procedure for administering emergency oxygen
- Outline the procedure for recording the blood pressure

CLINICAL SIGNS OF ACUTE ILLNESS

The clinical signs of acute illness and deterioration are usually similar regardless the underlying cause, because they reflect compromise of the respiratory, cardiovascular and neurological functions (Nolan *et al.*, 2005). These clinical signs are commonly:

- Tachypnoea (respiratory rate >20/minute): a particularly important indicator of an at-risk patient (Goldhill *et al.*, 1999) and is the most common abnormality found in acute illness (Goldhill & McNarry, 2004);

- Tachycardia (heart rate >100 beats per minute);

- Hypotension (usually a systolic blood pressure <90mmHg);

- Altered consciousness level (e.g. lethargy, confusion, restlessness or falling level of consciousness) (Resuscitation Council (UK), 2006b; Jevon & Ewens, 2007).

The identification of the clinical signs of acute illness (together with the patient's history, examination and appropriate investigations) is central to objectively identifying patients who are sick or deteriorating (Buist *et al.*, 1999). However, these clinical signs of deterioration are often subtle and can go unnoticed. It is therefore important to assess the patient following the systematic ABCDE approach.

THE ABCDE APPROACH

The Resuscitation Council (UK) (2006b) has issued guidance on the recognition and treatment of the sick patient. Adapted from the ALERT course (Smith, 2003), these guidelines follow the logical and systematic ABCDE approach to patient assessment:

- airway;

- breathing;

- circulation;

- disability;

- exposure.

When assessing the patient, undertake a complete initial assessment, identifying and treating life-threatening problems first, before moving on to the next part of assessment. The effectiveness of treatment/intervention should be evaluated, and regular reassessment undertaken. The need to call for an ambulance should be recognised and other members of the multidisciplinary team should be utilised as appropriate so that patient assessment, instigation of appropriate monitoring and interventions can be undertaken simultaneously.

Irrespective of their training, experience and expertise in clinical assessment and treatment, all dental professionals can follow the ABCDE approach; clinical skills, knowledge, expertise and local circumstances will determine what aspects of the assessment and treatment are undertaken.

GENERAL PRINCIPLES OF THE ABCDE APPROACH

The general principles of the ABCDE approach to assessing the sick patient are as follows:

- The ABCDE approach should be followed when both assessing and treating the patient.

- Life-threatening problems, once identified, should be treated before moving on to the next part of the assessment.

- If there is further deterioration, reassessment should be performed, starting with the airway.

- The effects of any treatment administered should be evaluated.

- The need for extra help, e.g. calling 999 for an ambulance, should be considered.

- All the members of the dental team should be involved, allowing essentials tasks such as collecting emergency equipment and oxygen or calling 999 for an ambulance to be undertaken simultaneously.

- Effective organisation and communication within the dental team are paramount.

- The initial aim of treatment is to keep the patient alive, prevent deterioration and ideally achieve clinical improvement; hopefully this will buy time while awaiting expert help and more definitive treatment.

- The ABCDE approach can be used by dental professionals irrespective of their training, expertise and experience in clinical assessment or treatment; individual experience and training will determine which aspects of assessment are undertaken and which treatments are administered.

- Basic interventions e.g. laying the patient flat or administering oxygen, are often all that are required (Resuscitation Council (UK), 2006b).

THE ABCDE APPROACH TO THE SICK PATIENT

Safety

Ensure the environment is safe and free of hazards and follow infection control guidelines e.g. wash hands, put on gloves if necessary.

Communication

Talk to the patient and evaluate his response: a normal response, indicates he has a clear airway, is breathing and has adequate cerebral perfusion; the inability to complete sentences could indicate extreme respiratory distress. An inappropriate response or no response could indicate an acute life-threatening physiological disturbance (Gwinnutt, 2006) e.g. inability to complete sentences in one breath is a severe adverse sign in a patient having an asthmatic attack (British Thoracic Society, 2008).

Patient's general appearance

Note the patient's general appearance, his colour and whether he appears content and relaxed or distressed and anxious.

Senior help

Request help from the senior dental practitioner. During the assessment process, consider whether it is necessary to call 999 for an ambulance.

Oxygen, emergency equipment/drugs

Ask a colleague to fetch the oxygen and other emergency equipment/drugs if required.

Monitoring devices

If one is available, attach a pulse oximeter (see page 33) (Resuscitation Council UK, 2006).

Airway

Assessment of airway

During the assessment of the airway, it is important to quickly establish if it is obstructed and treat it effectively. Look, listen and feel for the signs of airway obstruction. Partial airway obstruction will result in noisy breathing.

- *Gurgling:* indicates the presence of fluid, e.g. secretions or vomit, in the mouth or upper airway; usually seen in a patient with altered level of consciousness who is having difficulty or is unable to clear his own airway.

- *Snoring:* indicates that the pharynx is being partially obstructed by the tongue; usually seen in a patient with altered level of consciousness lying in a supine position.

- *Stridor:* high-pitched sound during inspiration, indicating partial upper airway obstruction; usually due to either a foreign body or laryngeal oedema.

- *Wheeze:* noisy musical whistling type sound due to the turbulent flow of air through narrowed bronchi and bronchioles, more pronounced on expiration; causes include asthma and chronic obstructive pulmonary disorder (COPD).

Complete airway obstruction can be detected by no air movement at the patient's mouth and nose. Paradoxical chest and abdominal movements ('see-saw' movement of the chest) may be observed and, if not rapidly treated, central cyanosis will develop (late sign of airway obstruction).

Treatment of airway obstruction

Airway obstruction is a medical emergency. If untreated, it can lead to hypoxia/hypoxaemia (low oxygen levels in the blood), which can damage the brain, kidneys and heart; cardiac arrest and even death could ensue (Resuscitation Council (UK), 2006b).

If the patient has airway obstruction, whether partial or complete, treat the underlying cause if possible. In most situations, simple interventions are sufficient to clear the airway. For example:

- Perform head tilt, chin lift to open the airway in an unconscious patient (see pages 130–1).

- Suction the pharynx if there is blood or vomit in it.

- Consider inserting an oropharyngeal airway to help keep a patent airway in an unconscious patient (see pages 133–6).

- Perform back slaps and abdominal thrusts as necessary if there is foreign body airway obstruction (see pages 145–8).

- Administer high concentration of oxygen via a non-rebreathe mask (Figure 3.1) (see pages 37–9) (Jevon & Ewens, 2007).

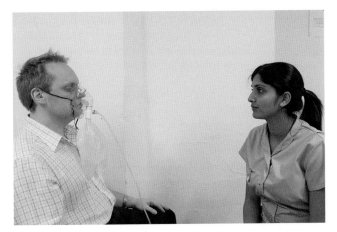

Figure 3.1 Administering high concentration of oxygen via a non-rebreathe mask.

Breathing

Assessment of breathing

During the assessment of breathing, it is important to quickly diagnose and treat any life-threatening breathing problems, e.g. acute asthma (Resuscitation Council (UK), 2006a). Follow the familiar 'look, listen and feel' approach to assess breathing:

- *Count the respiratory rate:* normal respiratory rate is 12–20/minute (Resuscitation Council (UK), 2006a). Tachypnoea (fast respiratory rate) is usually the first sign that the patient has respiratory distress (Smith, 2003). It is an indicator of illness, that the patient may deteriorate and that medical help is required (Resuscitation Council (UK), 2006b). Bradypnoea (slow respiratory rate) is an ominous sign and could indicate imminent respiratory arrest; causes include drugs, e.g. opiates, and fatigue.

- *Evaluate chest movement:* chest movement should be symmetrical; unilateral chest movement suggests unilateral pathology, e.g. pneumothorax, pneumonia, pleural effusion (Smith, 2003).

- *Evaluate the depth of breathing:* only marked degrees of hyperventilation and hypoventilation can be detected; hyperventilation may be seen if the patient is having a panic attack (Ford *et al.*, 2005).

- *Note the oxygen saturation (SaO₂) reading (if available):* the normal reading is usually 97–100%. A low SaO_2 could indicate respiratory distress or compromise.

- *Listen to the breathing:* normal breathing is quiet. Rattling airway noises indicate the presence of airway secretions, usually due to the patient being unable to cough sufficiently or unable to take a deep breath in (Smith, 2003). The presence of stridor or wheeze indicates partial, but significant, airway obstruction (see above).

Treatment of compromised breathing

If the patient has compromised breathing it is paramount to provide prompt effective treatment. In addition, during the initial assessment of breathing, it is essential to diagnose and effectively treat immediately life-threatening conditions, e.g. acute severe asthma (Resuscitation Council (UK), 2006). If the patient has compromised breathing:

- Position the patient in a upright position to help maximise chest movement; if he is in the dental chair, he may find it helpful to sit on the side of the chair with his legs down and feet touching the floor.

- Administer high concentration of oxygen via a non-rebreathe mask (Figure 3.1) (see pages 37–9) (Jevon & Ewens, 2007); If possible treat the underlying cause. In the dental practice the most likely cause of compromised breathing that could be treated is asthma, i.e. administer beta agonist inhaler (see page 50).

Circulation

Assessment of circulation

- *Count the pulse (radial or carotid):* a weak pulse suggests a poor cardiac output. In a vasovagal attack, the pulse is slow; in anaphylactic shock the pulse is fast.

- *Check the colour and temperature of the hands and fingers:* signs of cardio-vascular compromise include cool and pale peripheries.

- *Measure the capillary refill time (CRT):* holding a fingertip at the level of the heart, apply sufficient pressure for 5 seconds to cause blanching of the skin, and then release (Figure 3.2). Normal CRT is < 2 seconds; a prolonged CRT could indicate poor peripheral perfusion, though other causes can include cool ambient temperature, poor lighting and old age (Resuscitation Council UK, 2006b). A prolonged capillary refill time may be seen in anaphylaxis.

- *Measure the blood pressure:* a systolic BP < 90 mmHg suggests shock.

- *Establish if the patient has chest pain:* central crushing chest pain is suggestive of a heart attack (see pages 64–70.)

Figure 3.2 Measuring capillary refill time.

Treatment of a problem with circulation

The treatment of a problem with circulation will depend on the cause:

- *Low blood pressure due to a vasovagal episode or simple faint:* lay the patient flat with the legs raised (often, no other treatment is required) (see pages 72–4).

- *Anaphylactic shock:* lay the patient flat with the legs raised (unless this compromises breathing), administer high concentration of oxygen and administer adrenaline, while a colleague calls 999 for an ambulance.

- *Chest pain:* sit patient upright; treatment could include GTN spray, aspirin and high inspired concentration oxygen; it will usually be necessary to dial 999 for an ambulance.

- Administer high concentration of oxygen via a non-rebreathe mask if necessary (Figure 3.1) (see pages 37–9) (Jevon & Ewens, 2007).

Disability

Assessment of disability

To assess disability (central nervous system function):

- *Evaluate the patient's level of consciousness:* use the AVPU method and assign the patient as being **A** (alert), **V** (responds to a vocal stimulus), **P** (responds to a painful stimulus) or **U** (unresponsive to all stimuli) (Resuscitation Council (UK), 2006b) (Figure 3.3). Causes of altered level of consciousness include hypoxia, cerebral hypoperfusion due to low blood pressure, and recent administration of sedative or analgesic medications.

```
Alert
Responds to Voice
Responds to Pain
Unresponsive
```

Figure 3.3 AVPU: scale for assessing level of consciousness.

- *Examine the pupils:* compare size, equality and reaction to light of each pupil. Recent injection of an illicit drug (opiate) can cause pinpoint pupils.
- *Check the blood glucose:* if the patient has altered level of consciousness, check the blood glucose to exclude hypoglycaemia (see pages 98–9).
- *Check the patient's medication history:* is there a reversible drug-induced cause of altered level of consciousness?

Treatment of altered level of consciousness

- Review ABC to exclude hypoxia or low blood pressure as a cause of altered level of consciousness.
- Consider placing the patient in the lateral position to help protect the airway, particularly if unresponsive to all stimuli.
- Consider administering high concentration of oxygen via a non-rebreathe mask (Figure 3.1) (see pages 37–9) (Jevon & Ewens, 2007).
- If hypoglycaemia is suspected/confirmed, administer appropriate treatment to raise blood glucose levels (see pages 95–7).
- Consider the need to call 999 for an ambulance.

Exposure

In order to assess and treat the patient properly, it may be necessary to loosen or remove some of his clothes; his dignity should be respected and heat loss minimised (Resuscitation Council (UK), 2006b). If anaphylaxis is suspected, examine the skin for urticaria.

PRINCIPLES OF PULSE OXIMETRY

Some dental practices (usually those that administer sedation) will have access to a pulse oximeter (Figure 3.4). It will therefore be helpful to discuss the principles of pulse oximetry and oxygen saturation monitoring.

Figure 3.4 Pulse oximeter.

Pulse oximetry is widely regarded as one of the greatest advances in clinical monitoring (Giuliano & Higgins, 2005) since the invention of the ECG (Fox, 2002). It is a simple, non-invasive method of measuring arterial oxygen saturation (Higgins, 2005) expressed as SpO_2 (Welch, 2005). Pulse oximetry was developed in the 1980s; before this, oxygenation assessment was reliant on subjective and unreliable physical assessment of the skin for cyanosis (Giuliano & Higgins, 2005) which, when present, is an indicator of advanced hypoxaemia (Giuliano, 2006).

Pulse oximetry only measures the extent to which haemoglobin is saturated with oxygen and does not provide information on oxygen delivery to the tissues or ventilatory function (Higgins 2005). Nevertheless, it is an invaluable monitoring tool in a variety of clinical settings, including in the dental practice when sedation is being administered to the patient.

Role of pulse oximetry

Hypoxaemia can occur in patients in the dental practice, e.g. while sedated or during a severe asthma attack. If unrecognised and untreated, it can lead to cellular death and organ dysfunction.

Cyanosis is a late sign of hypoxaemia and the oxygen saturation must decrease to 80–85% before any changes in skin colour become apparent (Giuliano & Higgins, 2005). In addition, manifestations of hypoxaemia including restlessness, confusion, agitation, cyanosis, combative behaviour and tachycardia may be missed or wrongly interpreted (Technology Subcommittee of the Working Group on Critical Care, 1992).

Pulse oximetry, the fifth vital sign (Welch, 2005) will immediately alert the dental practitioner to a fall in arterial oxygen saturations and the development of hypoxaemia, prior to visual recognition of cyanosis. In clinical practice an oxygen saturation of less than 90% is of concern.

> The absence of cyanosis does not exclude severe hypoxaemia; it will not be present if the haemoglobin concentration is low or if there is poor perfusion of the capillaries

The mechanics of pulse oximetry

Pulse oximetry is a differential measurement based on the spectrophotometric absorption method using the Beer-Lambert Law for optical absorption (Welch, 2005).

The pulse oximeter probe consists of two light-emitting diodes (one red and one infrared) on one side of the probe. These transmit red and infrared light across the vascular bed, usually a finger tip or ear lobe, to a photodetector on the other side of the probe (Welch, 2005). The ratio of absorption is relative to the concentration of oxygenated haemoglobin to deoxygenated haemoglobin (Welch, 2005). The more oxygenated the blood is, more red light passes through and less infrared light passes through (Giuliano, 2006). By calculating the ratios of red to infrared light change over time, oxygen saturation is calculated (Guiliano, 2006).

Uses of pulse oximetry in the dental practice

Pulse oximetry is indicated in any clinical situation where hypoxaemia may occur. In the dental practice it could be used in patients receiving sedation and acutely ill patients, e.g. severe asthma attack.

Advantages of pulse oximetry

Pulse oximetry is an inexpensive, non-invasive and portable method of continuous measurement of arterial oxygen saturation which facilitates the early detection of hypoxaemia. It also provides information about the heart rate (Welch, 2005).

Normal values for oxygen saturation

The normal range for oxygen saturation measurements is >95% (Fox, 2002), though lower measurements may be 'normal' for some patients, e.g. those who have COPD (Fox, 2002).

RECOGNITION OF THE SICK PATIENT:
THE ABCDE APPROACH

Procedure for pulse oximetry

The following preliminary points should be observed (adapted from Jevon & Ewens, 2007).

- Ensure the probe is clean.

- Wash and dry hands.

- Explain the procedure to the patient.

- Select an appropriate site with an adequate pulsating vascular bed. Sites include finger (most popular) and ear lobe (less accurate); toes can be used instead of fingers, but this is generally not practical in the dental practice. In addition, poor perfusion is more common in the toes. If the finger is used, it is usual practice to remove any nail polish (Higgins, 2005) (obtain patient's consent first).

- Ensure that the trace is reliable and corresponds to pulse rate, i.e. oxygen saturation measurements are accurate.

- Ensure the alarms on the pulse oximeter are set within locally agreed limits and according to the patient's condition.

- Regularly monitor the patient's vital signs.

- Monitor the readings.

Causes of inaccuracy

Inaccurate readings can be caused by any of the factors listed below.

- *Carbon monoxide poisoning*: false high readings (Mathews, 2005).

- *Methaemglobinaemia* (changes in the structure of iron in haemoglobin) and if present in high doses can give false high or low readings (Welch, 2005).

- *Poor vascular perfusion*: pulse oximeter requires pulsatile blood flow to evaluate oxygen saturation.

- *Venous pulsation*: e.g. tricuspid valve failure, securing the probe too tightly (Fox, 2002; Welch, 2005), heart failure, inflating blood pressure cuff distal to the probe, resulting in a false low reading.

- *Poor vascular perfusion*: e.g. in hypotension, anaphylactic shock or peripheral vascular disease, resulting in a false low reading.

- *Cardiac arrhythmias* such as atrial fibrillation can cause inadequate and irregular perfusion, resulting in a false low reading.

- *Factors that affect light absorption*: skin pigmentation, dried blood and dark nail polish (Welch, 2005).

- *Bright external light*, particularly fluorescent lighting (Fox, 2002; Gwinnutt, 2006) can give a false high reading.

- *Anaemia.*

- *Patient on supplementary oxygen* can mean that hypoxaemia will not be detected early.

- *Patient movement*, e.g. shivering; though modern pulse oximeters can minimise the interference from patient movement (Gwinnutt, 2006).

Limitations

Although pulse oximetry measures oxygen saturation and can detect hypoxaemia, it does not provide an indication of the adequacy of ventilation and carbon dioxide retention. Davidson and Hosie (1993) reported a case of a postoperative patient who had a normal oxygen saturation (95%), but had abnormally high carbon dioxide levels causing a life-threatening respiratory acidosis. Failure to detect hypoventilation in a patient is an example of a false sense of security generated by a single physiological variable being within safe limits. It is therefore paramount that, when using pulse oximetry, the dental practitioner is aware of its limitations and always monitors the patient's vital signs following the ABCDE approach.

Trouble-shooting

It is important to ensure a reliable trace at all times. If it is difficult to secure an acceptable trace:

- warm and rub the skin to improve circulation;
- try a different probe site, e.g. ear lobe;
- try a different probe or a different pulse oximeter.

Complications

Pulse oximetry is very safe. Complications can occasionally occur, but generally only after prolonged use, which will not be the case in the dental practice.

PROCEDURE FOR ADMINISTERING OXYGEN TO THE ACUTELY ILL PATIENT

The non-rebreathing oxygen mask (Figure 3.1) enables the delivery of high concentrations of oxygen and is recommended for use in acutely ill patients (Resuscitation Council (UK), 2006a). To ensure the mask is functioning correctly and is effectively used, it is important to follow the manufacturer's recommendations for simple basic checks prior to use (Intersurgical, 2003).

Description

The non-rebreathing mask (sometimes called a Hudson mask) with an oxygen reservoir bag can be used to deliver high concentrations of oxygen to a spontaneously breathing patient. A one-way valve diverts the oxygen flow into the reservoir bag during expiration; the contents of the reservoir bag together with the high flow oxygen, results in minimal entrainment of air and an inspired oxygen concentration of approximately 85% (Gwinnutt, 2006). The valve also prevents the patient's exhaled gases from entering the reservoir bag. The use of the oxygen reservoir bag helps to increase the inspired oxygen concentration by preventing oxygen loss during inspiration.

It is important to ensure that a sufficient oxygen flow rate is used to ensure that the oxygen reservoir bag does not collapse during inspiration (Resuscitation Council (UK), 2006a). An oxygen flow rate of 12–15 litres/minute is recommended (Gwinnutt, 2006).

Procedure

- Ensure the patient is in an upright position to maximise breathing.

- If available in the dental practice, request that pulse oximetry is commenced.

- Explain the procedure to the patient.

- Attach the oxygen tubing to the oxygen source.

- Set the oxygen flow rate to 12–15 litres/min (Gwinnutt, 2006).

- Occlude the valve between the mask and the oxygen reservoir bag (Figure 3.5) and check that the reservoir bag is filling up. Remove the finger.

- Squeeze the oxygen reservoir bag (Figure 3.6) to check the patency of the valve between the mask and the reservoir bag. If the valve is working correctly it will be possible to empty the reservoir bag. If the reservoir bag does not empty, discard it and select another mask (Smith, 2003).

Figure 3.5 Checking the non-rebreathe mask: with oxygen 12–15 litres attached, occlude the valve between the mask and the oxygen reservoir bag, checking that the reservoir bag fills up.

Figure 3.6 Checking the non-rebreathe mask: with oxygen 12–15 litres attached, release the pressure on the valve and squeeze the oxygen reservoir bag – it should empty.

- Again occlude the valve between the mask and the oxygen reservoir bag, allowing the reservoir bag to fill up.

- Place the mask with a filled oxygen reservoir bag on the patient's face, ensuring a tight fit.

- Adjust the oxygen flow rate sufficient to ensure that the reservoir bag deflates by approximately one third with each breath (Smith, 2003).

Figure 3.7 Respiratory rate indictor.

- Provide reassurance to the patient.
- Closely monitor the patent's vital signs. In particular, assess the patient's response to the oxygen therapy, e.g. respiratory rate, mechanics of breathing, colour, oxygen saturation levels, level of consciousness.
- Discontinue or reduce the inspired oxygen concentration as appropriate following advice from the senior dental practitioner (Intersurgical, 2003).

Respiratory rate indicator

Some masks have a respiratory rate indicator (Figure 3.7) to help the healthcare practitioner to monitor the patient's respiratory rate. This indicator can be affected by:

- the patient's respiratory rate;
- the orientation of the indicator;
- the oxygen flow rate;
- the fit of the mask to the patient's face;
- the presence of moisture in the indicator tube – this can actually stop the indicator from working (Intersurgical, 2003).

The respiratory rate indicator should only be used as a guide and should not replace close monitoring of the patient's breathing

PROCEDURE FOR RECORDING BLOOD PRESSURE

Of all the measurements routinely undertaken in clinical practice, the recording of blood pressure is potentially the most unreliably and incorrectly performed measurement (British Hypertensive Society, 2006a). It is essential that blood pressure recordings are accurate and reliable: good practice can significantly reduce measurement errors and help ensure that the blood pressure recording obtained is accurate and reliable.

Systolic and diastolic blood pressure

Systolic blood pressure is peak blood pressure in the artery following ventricular systole (contraction). *Diastolic blood pressure* is the level to which the arterial blood pressure falls during ventricular diastole (relaxation) (Talley & O'Connor, 2001).

Korotkoff sounds

Five different sound phases known as 'Korotkoff sounds' (Korotkoff, a Russian surgeon, first described the auscultation method of measuring blood pressure in 1905) can be heard as the blood pressure cuff is slowly released:

- Phase 1: a thud;
- Phase 2: a blowing or swishing noise;
- Phase 3: a softer thud than in sound 1;
- Phase 4: a disappearing blowing noise;
- Phase 5: silence (Talley & O'Connor, 2001; Dougherty & Lister, 2008).

Practically, the systolic reading is when the Korotkoff sounds are first heard and the diastolic reading is when the sounds disappear (British Hypertensive Society, 2006a).

Which arm?

The blood pressure should initially be measured in both arms and the arm with the higher readings should be used for subsequent measurements (MHRA, 2006; NICE & British Hypertensive Society, 2006). Although a difference in blood pressure measurements between the arms can be expected in 20% of

Figure 3.8 Mercury sphygmomanometer.

patients, if this difference is >20 mmHg for systolic or >10 mmHg for diastolic on three consecutive readings, further investigation will probably be indicated (MHRA, 2006; NICE & British Hypertensive Society, 2006).

Procedure for manual measurement of a blood pressure

The traditional manual blood pressure device (Figure 3.8) using auscultation is still very popular, and when used correctly, a reliable method of recording blood pressure. The following procedure for its use is recommended.

- Ideally ensure that the patient has been resting for at least 5 minutes and is comfortably relaxed.

- Check the equipment, ensuring it is in good working order.

- Explain the procedure to the patient and obtain his consent.

- Ask the patient to remove any tight clothing from around his arm.

- Ensure the patient's arm is supported at the level of the heart. If the arm is unsupported, the blood pressure is likely to be erroneously increased due to muscle contraction in the arm (Smith, 2003). If the arm is higher than the level of the heart, this can lead to an underestimation of the diastolic pressure by as much as 10 mmHg (MHRA, 2006).

- Select an appropriately sized cuff: the bladder of the cuff should encircle at least 80% of the arm but no more than 100%.

- Place the cuff snugly onto the patient's arm, with the centre of the bladder over the brachial artery – most cuffs have a 'brachial artery indicator', an arrow which be aligned with the brachial artery.

- Position the manometer near to the patient. It should be vertical and at the practitioner's eye level.

- Ask the patient to refrain from talking as this can result in an inaccurate higher blood pressure.

- Estimate the systolic pressure: palpate the brachial artery, inflate the cuff and note the reading when the brachial pulse disappears. Then deflate the cuff.

- Inflate the cuff to 30 mmHg above the estimated systolic level, which was required to occlude the brachial pulse. Approximately 5% of the population has an auscultatory gap; this is when the Korotkoff sounds disappear just below the systolic pressure and reappear above the diastolic pressure (Talley & O'Connor, 2001). Estimating the systolic pressure will help ensure that the cuff is sufficiently inflated to record an accurate systolic pressure.

- Palpate the brachial artery.

- Place the diaphragm of the stethoscope gently over the brachial artery. Avoid applying excessive pressure on the diaphragm and don't tuck the diaphragm under the edge of the cuff because either of these actions could partially occlude the brachial artery, delaying the occurrence of the Korotoff sounds (Dougherty & Lister, 2004) (Figure 3.9).

- Open the valve and slowly deflate the cuff at a rate of 2–3 mm/sec, recording when the Korotkoff sounds first appear (systolic) and disappear (diastolic).

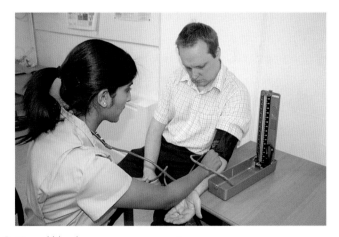

Figure 3.9 Manual blood pressure measurement.

- Document the systolic and diastolic blood pressure readings on the patient's observation chart following local protocols. Compare with previous readings and inform nurse in charge/medical team as appropriate.

(British Hypertensive Society 2006a,b; NICE & British Hypertensive Society, 2006)

Errors in blood pressure measurement

Errors in blood pressure measurement can occur for several reasons (British Hypertensive Society, 2006a) including:

- Defective equipment, e.g. leaking tubing or a faulty valve;
- Failure to ensure the mercury column reads 0 mmHg at rest;
- Too rapid deflation of the cuff;
- Use of incorrectly sized cuff: if it is too small the blood pressure will be overestimated and if it is too big the blood pressure will be underestimated;
- Cuff not at the same level as the heart;
- Failure to observe the mercury level properly – the top of the mercury column should be at eye level;
- Poor technique (e.g. failing to note when the sounds disappear);
- Digit preference, rounding the reading up to the nearest 5 or 10 mmHg;
- Observer bias, e.g. expecting a young patient's blood pressure to be normal.

Automated blood pressure devices

When automated blood pressure devices were first manufactured, their accuracy and reliability was questioned (Beevers et al., 2001). However, improved technology has led to the development of more accurate and reliable devices (Beevers et al., 2001), some of which have been tested and approved for use by the British Hypertensive Society (2006a).

Most automated devices measure blood pressure using one of the following techniques:

- oscillometry to detect arterial blood flow (most commonly used device);
- a microphone to detect the Korotkoff sounds;
- ultrasound to detect arterial blood flow (British Hypertensive Society, 2006a).

Procedure for automated measurement of blood pressure

The principles for the accurate measurement of blood pressure using an automated electronic device will be similar to the manual recording of blood pressure using a sphygmomanometer in respect of preparing the patient, positioning the patient, and choice and placement of cuff (Dougherty & Lister, 2004). However, when using an automated electronic device, it is important to be familiar with its working and to follow the manufacturer's recommendations when using it.

CONCLUSION

This chapter has provided an overview to the principles of recognition of the sick patient. The clinical signs of acute illness have been listed and the ABCDE approach has been discussed and described.

REFERENCES

Beevers G, Marshall T, Rouse A (2001) Blood pressure measurement part 1: sphygmomanometry: factors common to all techniques. *BMJ*; 322:981–985.

British Hypertensive Society (2006a) Blood pressure measurement with mercury blood pressure monitors (ww.bhsoc.org).

British Hypertensive Society (2006b) Let's Do It Well (www.bhsoc.org/pdfs/hit.pdf).

British Thoracic Society (2008) *2008 British Guideline on the Management of Asthma*. British Thoracic Society, London.

Buist M, Jarmolowski E, Burton P *et al.* (1999) Recognising clinical instability in hospital patients before cardiac arrest or unplanned admission to intensive care. *Medical Journal of Australia*; 171:22–25.

Davidson J, Hosie H (1993) Limitations of pulse oximetry: respiratory insufficiency – a failure of detection. *BMJ*; 307:372–373.

Dougherty L, Lister S (2008) *The Royal Marsden Hospital Manual of Clinical Nursing Procedures*, 7th edn. Blackwell Publishing, Oxford.

Ford M, Hennessey I, Japp A (2005) *Introduction to Clinical Examination*. Elsevier, Oxford.

Fox N (2002) Pulse oximetry. *Nursing Times*; 98(40): 65–67.

Goldhill DR, Worthington L, Mulcahy A *et al.* (1999) The patient-at-risk team: identifying and managing seriously ill patients. *Anaesthesia*; 54:853–860.

Goldhill D, McNarry A (2004) Physiological abnormalities in early warning scores are related to mortality in adult inpatients. *British Journal of Anaesthesia*; 92(6):882–884.

Giuliano K, Higgins T (2005) New-generation pulse oximetry in the care of critically ill patients. *American Journal of Critical Care*; 14:26–37.

Guiliano K (2006) Knowledge of pulse oximetry among critical care nurses. *Dimensions of Critical Care Nursing*; 25(1):44–49.

Gwinnutt C (2006) *Clinical Anaesthesia*, 2nd edn. Blackwell Publishing, Oxford.

Higgins D (2005) Oxygen therapy. *Nursing Times*; 101(4):30–31.

Intersurgical (2003) *Non-rebreathing mask product literature.* Intersurgical, Wokingham.

Jevon P, Ewens B (2007) *Monitoring the Critically Ill Patient*, 2nd edn. Blackwell Publishing, Oxford.

Mathews P (2005) The latest in respiratory care. *Nursing Management supplement: critical care choices*; 18:20–21.

MHRA (2005) *Report of the Independent Advisory Group on Blood Pressure Monitoring in Clinical Practice.* Medicine and Healthcare products Regulatory Agency, London.

NICE & the British Hypertensive Society (2006) *NICE/BHS Hypertension Guideline Review* 28 June 2006 (www.bhsoc.org/NICE_BHS_Guidelines.stm).

Nolan J, Deakin C, Soar J *et al.* (2005) European Resuscitation Council Guidelines for Resuscitation 2005: Section 4. Adult advanced life support. *Resuscitation*; 67SS, S39-S86.

Resuscitation Council (UK) (2006a) *Medical emergencies and resuscitation standards for clinical practice and training for dental practitioners and dental care professionals in general dental practice.* Resuscitation Council (UK), London.

Resuscitation Council (UK) (2006b) *Advanced Life Support*, 5th edn. Resuscitation Council (UK), London.

Smith G (2003) *ALERT: Acute life-threatening events recognition and treatment*, 2nd edn. University of Portsmouth, Portsmouth.

Talley N, O'Connor S (2001) *Clinical Examination: A systematic guide to physical diagnosis.* Blackwell Science, Oxford.

Technology Subcommittee of the Working Group on Critical Care (1992) Non-invasive gas monitoring: a review for use in the adult critical care unit. *Canadian Medical Association Journal*; 146:703–712.

Welch J (2005) Pulse oximeters. *Biomedical Instrumentation and Technology*; March/April: 125–130.

Chapter 4

Respiratory disorders

INTRODUCTION

In the UK, 20% of all deaths are caused by respiratory disorders; in 2004, 117,000 deaths were caused by respiratory disease compared to 106,000 deaths from ischaemic heart disease (British Thoracic Society, 2006). Mortality rates from respiratory disease have changed little over the last two decades (British Thoracic Society, 2006). Social class inequality is estimated to be associated with 44% of all deaths from respiratory disease (British Thoracic Society, 2006).

The common occurrence of respiratory disease in the UK guarantees that it will be encountered in the dental practice. If serious, it can be life threatening. It is essential important to assess the patient following the ABCDE approach described in chapter 3.

The aim of this chapter is to understand the management of respiratory disorders.

LEARNING OUTCOMES

At the end of the chapter the reader will be able to:

- Discuss the management of an acute asthma attack
- Discuss the management of hyperventilation
- Discuss the management of exacerbation of chronic obstructive pulmonary disease
- Describe the procedure for using an inhaler device
- Describe the procedure for using a spacer device

MANAGEMENT OF ACUTE ASTHMA ATTACK

There is no a standard definition of asthma, though central to all definitions is the presence of key characteristics of the disease, i.e. one or more of wheeze, breathlessness, chest tightness and cough (British Thoracic Society, 2008).

There is considerable variation between patients in respect of the severity of episodes they experience and the overall course of the disease; for some patients their illness is well controlled and they are asymptomatic between acute attacks while for others the illness can progress to a state of irreversible airway obstruction (Bourke, 2003).

Incidence

It is estimated that in the UK 5.2 million people have asthma, of whom 1.1 million are children and 4.1 million are adults (Asthma UK, 2007). Although the number of children with asthma has fallen since a peak in the 1990s, the number of adults with asthma has risen with an increase of 400,000 between 2001 and 2004.

In the UK in 2002, 69,000 hospital admissions and 1400 deaths were attributed to asthma (Asthma UK, 2007). Although the incidence of acute asthma episodes in primary care is on the decline (Sunderland & Fleming, 2004), it is nevertheless important to be vigilant. Asthma related-emergencies account for 5% of all medical emergencies encountered in the dental practice (Müller *et al.*, 2008).

Pathogenesis

Asthma is characterised by episodes of reversible airway obstruction where hypersensitivity to certain triggers sets off an inflammatory response during which mucus is released and the muscles of the bronchi constrict (Deacon, 2008). The inflammatory process involves infiltration of the airway walls by various immune cells, oedema, hypertrophy of mucus glands and damage to the airway epithelial wall (Deacon, 2008). This airway remodelling from persistent inflammation can lead to permanent fibrotic damage.

Causes

Causes of an asthma attack include:

- smoking;
- dust;

RESPIRATORY DISORDERS

- animals;

- stress;

- chest infection.
  (Asthma UK, 2007).

In the dental practice, stress can trigger an acute asthma attack (Müller *et al.*, 2008).

Signs and symptoms

Signs and symptoms of asthma include:

- wheeze;

- shortness of breath;

- chest tightness;

- cough.
  (British Thoracic Society, 2008).

The hallmark of asthma is that these symptoms tend to be:

- variable;

- intermittent;

- worse at night;

- provoked by triggers including stress.
  (Jevon, 2006).

The speed of onset of an acute asthma attack can vary; although there is normally a history of deterioration over a period of days or weeks, an attack can sometimes occur suddenly with rapid deterioratation (Rees & Kanabar, 2007).

The severity of acute asthma can range from moderate to life threatening (Figure 4.1) (British Thoracic Society, 2008).

Patients with severe or life-threatening asthma may not be distressed; they could be quiet and drowsy (pre-cardiopulmonary arrest situation)

RESPIRATORY DISORDERS

RESPIRATORY DISORDERS

Management of acute severe asthma in adults in general practice

Many deaths from asthma are preventable. Delay can be fatal. Factors leading to poor outcome include:

- Clinical staff. Failing to assess severity by objective measurement
- Patients or relatives failing to appreciate severity
- Under-use of corticosteroids

Regard each emergency asthma consultation as for acute severe asthma until shown otherwise.

Assess and record:

- Peak expiratory flow (PEF)
- Symptoms and response to self treatment
- Heart and respiratory rates
- Oxygen saturation (by pulse oximetry, if available)

Caution: Patients with severe or life-threatening attacks may not be distressed and may not have all the abnormalities listed below. The presence of any should alert the doctor.

Moderate asthma	Acute severe asthma	Life-threatening asthma

INITIAL ASSESSMENT

PEF>50% best or predicted	PEF 33-50% best or predicted	PEF<33% best or predicted

FURTHER ASSESSMENT

■ Speech normal ■ Respiration <25 breaths/min ■ Pulse <110 beats/min	■ Can't complete sentences ■ Respiration ≥25 breaths/min ■ Pulse ≥110 beats/min	■ SpO$_2$ <92% ■ Silent chest, cyanosis or feeble respiratory effort ■ Bradycardia, dysrhythmia or hypotension ■ Exhaustion, confusion or coma

MANAGEMENT

Treat at home or in surgery and ASSESS RESPONSE TO TREATMENT	Consider admission	Arrange immediate ADMISSION

TREATMENT

■ High-dose β$_2$ bronchodilator:
  - Via oxygen-driven nebuliser (salbutamol 5 mg or terbutaline 10 mg)
  - Or via spacer (4-10 puffs [given one at a time single puffs, tidal breathing and inhaled separately] repeated at intervals of 10-20 minutes) or air-driven nebuliser
If PEF >50-75% predicted/best:
■ Give prednisolone 40-50 mg
■ Continue or step up usual treatment
If good response to first nebulised treatment *(symptoms improved, respiration and pulse settling and PEF >50%) continue or step up usual treatment and continue prednisolone*
	■ Oxygen 40-60% if available
	■ High-dose β$_2$ bronchodilator:
	  - Via oxygen-driven nebuliser (salbutamol 5 mg or terbutaline 10 mg)
	  - Or via spacer (4-10 puffs [given one at a time single puffs, tidal breathing and inhaled separately] repeated at intervals of 10-20 minutes)
	■ Prednisolone 40-50 mg or IV hydrocortisone 100 mg
	■ **If no response in acute severe asthma: ADMIT**
		■ Oxygen 40-60%
		■ Prednisolone 40-50 mg or IV hydrocortisone 100 mg immediately
		■ High dose β$_2$ bronchodilator and ipratropium:
		  - Via oxygen-driven nebuliser (salbutamol 5 mg or terbutaline 10 mg) and ipratropium 0.5mg)
		  - Or via spacer (4-10 puffs [given one at a time single puffs, tidal breathing and inhaled separately] repeated at intervals of 10-20 minutes)

Admit to hospital if any: ■ life-threatening features ■ features of acute severe asthma present after initial treatment ■ previous near-fatal asthma Lower threshold for admission if **afternoon or evening attack, recent nocturnal symptoms or hospital admission, previous severe attacks, patient unable to assess own condition, or concern over social circumstances.**	**If admitting the patient to hospital:** ■ Stay with patient until ambulance arrives ■ Send written asssessment and referral details to hospital ■ Give high-dose β$_2$ bronchodilator via oxygen-driven nebuliser in ambulance	**Follow up after treatment or discharge from hospital:** ■ **GP review within 48 hours** ■ Monitor symptoms and PEF ■ Check inhaler technique ■ Written asthma action plan ■ Modify treatment according to guidelines for chronic persistent asthma ■ Address potentially preventable contributors to admission

Figure 4.1 British Thoracic Society (2008) guidelines on the management of acute asthma. Reproduced with kind permission.

Figure 4.2 Example of a short-acting beta-2 adrenoceptor stimulant inhaler.

Treatment

The British Thoracic Society has issued guidelines on the management of acute asthma (Figure 4.1).

- Assess the patient following the ABCDE approach described in chapter 3.

- Sit the patient up (Ramrakha & Moore, 2004).

- If available, consult the patient's individual action plan in the event of an asthma attack (British Thoracic Society, 2008).

- Encourage the patient to take two puffs of a short-acting beta-2 adrenoceptor stimulant inhaler, e.g. salbutamol (100 μg/puff) (Figure 4.2) (British Medical Association & Royal Pharmaceutical Society, 2008). Hopefully the patient will be using his own inhaler and should therefore be familiar with its use and will be administering what his own general practitioner has prescribed. However, if he doesn't have this with him, use the inhaler stored in the emergency drugs box in the dental practice. (The correct procedure for using an inhaler is described on pages 57–9.)

- If the patient doesn't rapidly respond, administer further puffs (British Medical Association & Royal Pharmaceutical Society, 2008).

- If the patient is unable to take his inhaler effectively, administer further puffs through a spacer device (Figure 4.3) (see pages 59–62); if one is not available, a plastic or paper cup with a hole in the bottom for the inhaler

Figure 4.3 Spacer device.

Figure 4.4 Spacer device not available: a plastic or paper cup with a hole in the bottom for the inhaler mouthpiece will suffice (British Medical Association and Pharmaceutical Society of Great Britain, 2008).

mouthpiece will suffice (Figure 4.4) (British Medical Association & Royal Pharmaceutical Society, 2008).

- If the patient doesn't respond satisfactorily or if deterioration occurs, call 999 for an ambulance; while awaiting transfer to hospital, administer oxygen and also salbutamol 2.5–5 mg via a nebuliser (if this is not available, administer 4–10 puffs of salbutamol 100 μg/puff inhaler preferably via a large volume spacer device, repeating every 20 minutes if necessary (British Medical Association & Royal Pharmaceutical Society, 2008).

- Monitor the patient following the ABCDE approach, with particular attention to respiratory rate, heart rate and level of consciousness as tachypnoea, tachycardia and drowsiness are hallmarks of severe to life-threatening asthma (British Thoracic Society, 2008).

- Reassure the patient; an acute asthma attack is frightening and the need to be admitted to hospital can increase anxiety and exacerbate symptoms (Rees & Kanabar, 2007).

(Jevon, 2006; British Medical Association & Royal Pharmaceutical Society, 2008; British Thoracic Society, 2008)

Indications for hospital admission

Asthma has been classified into moderate, severe and life (British Thoracic Society, 2008) (Figure 4.1). For moderate, severe and life-threatening asthma, the following is recommended:

- *Moderate asthma:* treat at home or in the surgery and assess response to treatment;
- *Severe asthma:* immediate transfer to hospital should be arranged if the casualty is not responding to treatment;
- *Life-threatening asthma:* immediate transfer to hospital should be arranged (Resuscitation Council UK, 2006; British Thoracic Society, 2008).

Factors lowering the threshold for hospital admission include:

- Afternoon or evening episode;
- Recent nocturnal symptoms;
- Recent admission to hospital;
- Previous severe episodes;
- Patient unable to assess own condition;
- Concern regarding the patient's social circumstances.
  (British Thoracic Society, 2008; Rees & Kanabar, 2007).

Factors that contribute to a poor outcome

Factors that contribute to a poor outcome include:

- Healthcare practitioners failing to assess severity by objective measurement;
- Patients or relatives failing to recognise the severity of an attack;
- Under-use of corticosteroids.
  (British Thoracic Society, 2008).

Most deaths caused by asthma are preventable, but delay in referring the patient to hospital could be fatal (British Thoracic Society, 2008). Mortality is usually associated with failure to appreciate the severity of the exacerbation, leading to inadequate emergency treatment and delay in referring to hospital (British Thoracic Society, 2008).

MANAGEMENT OF HYPERVENTILATION

Hyperventilation can be defined as a fast respiratory rate resulting in an increased loss of carbon dioxide (Soanes & Stevenson, 2006). It is usually anxiety induced and may accompany a panic attack (Jevon, 2006). It can occur in a susceptible person who has recently experienced emotional or psychological trauma (St John Ambulance et al., 2006) and is not uncommon in the dental practice. It may be associated with attention-seeking behaviour.

Hyperventilation can lead to hypocapnia (low carbon dioxide levels in the blood) causing tingling in the extremities and the mouth, dizziness, trembling and cramps. Sometimes it can be mistaken for anaphylaxis (Resuscitation Council (UK), 2008), particularly if the patient starts to hyperventilate following the administration of a local anaesthetic. It is therefore always important to carefully assess the patient following the ABCDE approach so that serious illness can be excluded.

Treatment

- Reassure the patient; it may be necessary to be firm;
- If possible remove the cause of the distress or anxiety;
- If possible take the patient somewhere private where he can regain control of his breathing again (St John Ambulance et al., 2006).

If the patient is still hyperventilating despite the above, ask him to breathe into a paper bag:

- Ensure the paper bag covers both his nose and mouth (Figure 4.5);
- Ask him to breathe in and out slowly about 10 times;
- Then ask him to breath without the paper bag for 15 seconds;
- Alternate this cycle of breathing until the hyperventilation has stopped (St John Ambulance et al., 2006).

Figure 4.5 Management of hyperventilation: paper bag technique.

MANAGEMENT OF EXACERBATION OF CHRONIC OBSTRUCTIVE PULMONARY DISEASE

Chronic obstructive pulmonary disease (COPD) describes a spectrum of disease processes characterised by a chronic and progressive reduction in airflow (Deacon, 2008). Certain diseases, e.g. chronic bronchitis and emphysema, can cause COPD. In the dental practice a patient could have an exacerbation of COPD leading to acute breathlessness.

Incidence

Over 600,000 people in the UK have been diagnosed with COPD (a prevalence of 1%) (Calverly & Bellamy, 2000). Socioeconomic factors play a strong role in COPD: men aged 20–64 years who work in manual unskilled jobs are 14 times more likely to die from COPD than those in professional jobs (British Thoracic Society, 2006).

Causes

Cigarette smoking is the single most important risk factor for COPD (British Thoracic Society, 2008).

Clinical features

There is great variability in the symptoms experienced by patients with different severities of airflow obstruction and in the rate of disease progression (Deacon, 2008). However, the key clinical features are cough, wheeze and breathlessness (Halpin, 2003). A productive cough is common.

RESPIRATORY DISORDERS

Treatment

If a patient with COPD presents with acute shortness of breath in the dental practice:

- Assess the patient following the ABCDE approach described in chapter 3.

- Ensure the patient has a clear airway.

- Sit the patient in an upright position and administer oxygen. All critically ill patients should receive oxygen, even COPD patients in whom high concentrations of oxygen may depress breathing; these patients will sustain organ damage or cardiac arrest if their blood oxygen tensions are allowed to fall; the aim in this group of patients is to achieve a lower than normal PaO_2 (e.g. 8 kPa) or oxygen concentration (e.g. 90–92%) (Resuscitation Council (UK), 2006).

- If available, commence pulse oximetry.

- If indicated, encourage the patient to take two puffs of a short acting beta 2 adrenoceptor stimulant inhaler e.g. salbutamol (100 µg/puff) (Figure 4.2) (National Institute for Clinical Excellence, 2004).

- Monitor the patient's level of consciousness using the AVPU scale (page 32); if the patient's level of consciousness starts to deteriorate, e.g. he becomes drowsy, this is an adverse sign because it may indicate that he is becoming hypoxic and/or hypercapnoeic (rising levels of carbon dioxide).

- Consider the need to dial 999 for an ambulance.

PROCEDURE FOR USING AN INHALER

An inhaler is a device for the administration of an inhalation (McFerran & Martin, 2003). Various inhalers and formulations have been developed to help ensure the efficient delivery of drugs, simply and with minimal side effects (Rees & Kanabar, 2007). Various different devices are available, the most common being the pressurized metered dose inhaler (pMDI) (Figure 4.2). This type is available in most emergency drug boxes in dental practices. For the purpose of this book, the term inhaler will suffice.

Types of inhaler

Pressurized metered dose inhalers (pMDI) (Figure 4.2) are the commonest type of inhaler used. They are small, convenient, easy to carry and deliver a wide range of medications (Newell & Hume, 2006). However, the correct technique for using a pMDI can be difficult to master because it requires co-ordinating actuation and inhalation efficiently, and inhaling at the correct inspiratory flow rate (Pearce, 2000).

Some patients, particularly the elderly and small children, find it difficult to use a pMDI (British Medical Association & Royal Pharmaceutical Society, 2006). Patients with arthritis may also struggle to use them correctly (Rees & Kanabar, 2007). The use of the pMDI should therefore be reserved for patients who can consistently demonstrate that they can use them correctly (Pearce, 2000). Except for the Seretide Evohaler, the pMDI does not have a dose counter and some users require to estimate when it is nearly empty (Newell & Hume, 2006).

Breath-actuated inhalers (*Autohaler* and *Easi-Breathe*) are also small and easy to carry. As inhalation on the mouthpiece triggers the dose of medication to be released, they do not require the user to co-ordinate actuation and inhalation, which is an obvious advantage over pMDIs (Newell & Hume, 2006).

Dry powder inhalers (e.g. Accuhaler, Diskhaler) deliver the inhaled medication in the form of a dry powder. They are activated by the patient's inspiratory effort, thus automatically actuating the device (Newell & Hume, 2006). Although they are popular and generally easy to use, some devices require a fairly high respiratory flow rate in order to be activated (Newell & Hume, 2006).

Drugs administered using an inhaler

Drugs that can be administered using an inhaler include (Currie & Douglas, 2007):

- *Short-acting beta-2 agonists, e.g. salbutamol*: act on beta-2 adrenoreceptors in bronchial smooth muscle causing bronchodilation, which improves lung function and reduces breathlessness; effective for up to 6 hours. The Resuscitation Council (UK) recommends that a salbutamol inhaler should be kept in the dental practice (Resuscitation Council (UK), 2006).

- *Short-acting anticholinergics, e.g. ipratropium*: inhibit the action of acetylcholine resulting in relaxation of smooth muscle and bronchidilation, which improves lung function and reduces breathlessness; effective for up to 6 hours.

- *Long-acting beta-2 agonists, e.g. salmeterol*: effective for up to 12 hours.

- *Long-acting anticolinergics, e.g. tiotropium*: effective for up to 24 hours.

Drug delivery using an inhaler

An inhaler is designed to deliver the correct dose of an inhalation to an appropriate part of the airway. Even when an inhaler is used properly, only 10% of the drug reaches the airways below the larynx; 50% is deposited in the mouth with close to 90% eventually being swallowed (Currie & Douglas, 2007; Rees & Kanabar, 2007).

Procedure

The procedure for the use of a inhaler, the commonest inhaler and the one usually available in the dental practice's emergency drugs box, will now be described (Pearce, 2000; Jevon & Humphrey, 2007a; Currie & Douglas, 2007).

- Explain the procedure to the patient.
- Ask the patient to remove the mouthpiece cover from the inhaler (Figure 4.6).
- Ask the patient to shake the metered-dose inhaler and then breathe out.
- Advise the patient to place the mouthpiece into his mouth and to close his lips and teeth around it.
- At the start of inspiration, ask the patient to press the canister down while he continues to inhale slowly and deeply (Figure 4.7).
- Advise the patient to remove the mouthpiece from his mouth and to then close his lips.

Figure 4.6 Using an inhaler: remove the mouthpiece cover from the inhaler.

RESPIRATORY DISORDERS

Figure 4.7 Using an inhaler: at the start of inspiration, ask the patient to press the canister down while he continues to inhale slowly and deeply.

Figure 4.8 Using an inhaler: ask the patient to hold his breath for up to 10 seconds and then to breathe out normally.

- Ask the patient to hold his breath for up to 10 seconds and then to breathe out normally (Figure 4.8).
- If a second dose is required, wait 30–60 seconds and repeat the above steps before replacing the cover.
- Document that the inhaler has been administered.
- The use of the inhaler with a spacer device is recommended for some patients.

Procedures for using other inhalers

It is not possible to describe the use of all the different inhalers currently available. It is important to refer to the manufacturers' recommendations for the correct use of their inhalers.

Teaching and monitoring the patient

The patient should be carefully instructed on how to use his inhaler and it is important to ensure that he continues to use it correctly because inadequate inhalation technique may be mistaken for a lack of response to the prescribed drug (British Medical Association & Royal Pharmaceutical Society, 2008). Asthma UK's website contains detailed advice on how to correctly use inhalers which the patient may find helpful: www.asthma.org.uk

PROCEDURE FOR USING A SPACER DEVICE

A spacer device is a large plastic or metal container, with a mouthpiece at one end and a hole for the aerosol inhaler at the other (Asthma UK, 2007). It is basically a chamber that acts as a reservoir for the aerosol cloud, removing the need for co-ordinating actuation of a pMDI and inhalation (Pearce, 2000).

A spacer device will only work with an aerosol inhaler (Asthma UK, 2007). When used correctly, an inhaler with a spacer device attached is at least as effective as any other device for delivering inhaled drugs (Currie & Douglas, 2007).

Types of spacer device

Several spacer devices are currently available; the larger ones with a one-way valve, e.g. Nebuhaler Volumatic, are the most effective (British Medical Association & Royal Pharmaceutical Society, 2008).

Advantages of using a spacer device

Advantages of using a spacer device include:

- making aerosol inhalers easier to use: removes the need for co-ordination between actuation of an inhaler and inhalation;
- reducing the velocity of the aerosol and subsequent impaction on the patient's oropharynx;

- allowing more time for the propellant to evaporate, thus enabling a larger proportion of the drug particles to be inhaled and deposited in the lungs;
- reducing the risk of side effects from the higher doses of preventer medicines by reducing the amount of medicine that is swallowed and absorbed into the body (British Medical Association & Royal Pharmaceutical Society, 2008; Asthma UK, 2007).

Indications

Indications for using a spacer device include:

- patients with poor inhaler technique;
- children and infants;
- patients requiring high doses of medications.

Principles of using a spacer

- The spacer should be compatible with the inhaler that is being used;
- The drug should be administered by repeated single actuations of the metered dose inhaler into the spacer, each followed by an inhalation;
- There should be minimal delay between inhaler actuation and inhalation;
- Tidal breathing is just as effective as single breaths (British Thoracic Society, 2008).

Procedure

- Ensure the space device is compatible to the inhaler being used.
- If necessary, assemble the spacer device (some devices come in two halves) (Figure 4.9).
- Shake the inhaler.
- Remove the cap from the mouthpiece on the MDI and fit the MDI to the spacer device (Figure 4.10).
- Close lips and teeth around mouthpiece.
- Actuate the MDI.

(a)   (b)

Figure 4.9 (a), (b) Using a spacer device: assemble if necessary.

Figure 4.10 Using a spacer device: remove the cap from the mouthpiece on the inhaler and fit the latter to the spacer device.

- Inhale deeply and slowly; ask the patient to hold his breath for 10 seconds (or as long as it is comfortable) – inhalation should be as soon as possible following actuation, definitely within 30 seconds (Rees & Kanabar, 2007) (Figure 4.11).

- Remove the device from the mouth and close lips.

- Breathe out slowly (Asthma UK, 2007). It is recommended to take at least two deeply held breaths for each puff of the inhaler (Asthma UK, 2007). Some patients may find it difficult to take deep breaths – normal tidal breathing is considered just as effective (Asthma UK, 2007).

- If a second dose is required, wait 30–60 seconds before repeating the above procedure (Pearce, 2000).

RESPIRATORY DISORDERS

Figure 4.11 Using a spacer device: ask the patient to inhale deeply and slowly, then hold his breath for 10 seconds (or as long as it is comfortable).

- In infants and children under 2 years of age, attach a mask to the spacer device to facilitate its effective use; also hold the spacer at an angle of 45 degrees to keep the valve open – the medication can then be inhaled during normal tidal breathing (Rees & Kanabar, 2007).

(Jevon & Humphrey, 2007b)

CONCLUSION

Respiratory disorders can occur in the dental practice. In this chapter the management of an acute asthma attack, hyperventilation and exacerbation of chronic obstructive pulmonary disease have been discussed. In addition, the procedures for using an inhaler device and a spacer device have been described.

REFERENCES

Asthma UK (2007) www.asthma.org.uk (accessed 29 January 2009).
British Medical Association & Royal Pharmaceutical Society of Great Britain (2008) *British National Formulary 56*. BMJ Publishing, London.
British Thoracic Society (2006) *The Burden of Lung Disease*, 2nd edn. British Thoracic Society, London.
British Thoracic Society (2008) *2008 British Guideline on the Management of Asthma*. British Thoracic Society, London.
Bourke SJ (2003) *Respiratory Medicine*, 6th edn. Blackwell Publishing, Oxford.

Calverly P & Bellamy D (2000) The challenge of providing better care for patients with chronic obstructive pulmonary disease: the poor relation of airways obstruction? *Thorax*; 55(1):78–82.

Currie G, Douglas J (2007) Oxygen and inhalers. In Currie G (ed.) *ABC of COPD*, Blackwell Publishing, Oxford.

Deacon K (2008) Respiratory emergencies. In Jevon P *et al.* (eds) *Nursing Medical Emergency Patients*. Wiley-Blackwell, Oxford.

Halpin DMG (2003) *Your Questions Answered – COPD*. Churchill Livingstone, Edinburgh.

Jevon P (2006) *Emergency Care & First Aid for Nurses*. Elsevier, Oxford.

Jevon P, Humphrey N (2007a) Respiratory procedures part 5: use of an inhaler. *Nursing Times*; 103(36):24–25.

Jevon P, Humphrey N (2007b) Respiratory procedures part 4: use of a spacer device. *Nursing Times*; 103(35):24–25.

McFerran T, Martin E (2003) *Mini-Dictionary for Nurses*, 5th edn. Oxford University Press, Oxford.

Müller M, Hänsel M, Stehr S *et al.* (2008) A state-wide survey of medical emergency management in dental practices: incidence of emergencies and training experience. *Emergency Medicine Journal*; 25;296–300.

Newell K, Hume S (2006) Choosing the right inhaler for patients with asthma. *Nursing Standard*; 21(5):46–48.

National Institute for Clinical Excellence (2004) *Chronic obstructive pulmonary disease – Management of chronic obstructive pulmonary disease in adults in primary and secondary care*. NICE, London.

Pearce L (2000) Know How: Inhaler devices. *Nursing Times*; 96(16).

Ramrakha P, Moore K (2004) *Oxford Handbook of Acute Medicine*. Oxford University Press, Oxford.

Rees J, Kanabar D (2007) *ABC of Asthma*, 5th edn. Blackwell Publishing, Oxford.

Resuscitation Council (UK) (2006) *Medical emergencies and resuscitation standards for clinical practice and training for dental practitioners and dental care professionals in general dental practice*. Resuscitation Council (UK), London.

St John Ambulance, St Andrew's Ambulance, British Red Cross (2006) *First Aid Manual*, 9th edn. Dorling Kindersley, London.

Soanes C, Stevenson A (2006) *Oxford Dictionary of English*, 2nd edn. Oxford University Press, Oxford.

Sunderland R, Fleming M (2004) Continuing decline in acute asthma episodes in the community. *Archives of Disease in Childhood*; 89:282–285.

RESPIRATORY DISORDERS

Chapter 5

Cardiac disorders

INTRODUCTION

Coronary heart disease (CHD) is the leading cause of death in the UK (British Heart Foundation, 2009). Each year approximately 146,000 people suffer a myocardial infarction (MI; heart attack); one in three of these die before reaching hospital (British Heart Foundation, 2009). Chest pain, a characteristic symptom of CHD, is the commonest reason for alerting the emergency services; 10% of casualties taken to hospital with chest pain have had an acute myocardial infarction (Laird *et al.*, 2004).

The aim of this chapter is to understand the management of cardiac disorders.

LEARNING OUTCOMES

At the end of the chapter the reader will be able to:

- Discuss the management of angina
- Discuss the management of a myocardial infarction
- Discuss the management of palpitations
- Outlines the management of syncope

MANAGEMENT OF ANGINA

Angina pectoris is a condition marked by severe chest pain, often also spreading to the shoulders, arms and neck owing to an inadequate blood supply to the heart (from Latin *pectoris* meaning 'of the chest'; Soanes & Stevenson, 2006).

Angina occurs when an increased myocardial oxygen demand can not be met by the coronary blood supply (Wyatt *et al.*, 2006). There is usually a history of angina and risk factors include smoking, hypercholesterolaemia, hypertension, diabetes mellitus or a family history of ischaemic heart disease under the age of 60 years (Laird *et al.*, 2004).

If an angina attack occurs and not a myocardial infarction or heart attack (see below), the pain should ease with rest though the administration of glyceryl trinitrate spray or tablets may be needed. Hospital admission is not necessary if the symptoms are mild and resolve with the patient's own medication (British Medical Association & Royal Pharmaceutical Society, 2008).

Precipitants

Precipitants of angina include:

- exercise, particularly climbing stairs or an incline;
- emotion, particularly anger or anxiety;
- a large meal – can increase cardiac output by 20%;
- cold, windy weather;
- exciting programmes on television – 'match of the day' angina;
- life-like, frightening dreams;
- sexual intercourse, particularly if extramarital or with a new partner. (British Heart Foundation, 2009).

In the dental practice, a patient with a history of angina could develop angina if he has to walk up some stairs to the surgery or if he is very stressed about having dental treatment.

Signs and symptoms

- A crushing pain, heaviness or tightness in the chest; or
- A pain in the arm, throat, neck, jaw, back or stomach;
- Sometimes the pain is associated with sweating, light-headedness, sickness or becoming short of breath (British Heart Foundation, 2009).

Treatment

If the patient has not been diagnosed with heart disease and has chest pain, it is recommended to call 999 immediately (British Heart Foundation, 2009)

If a patient, who has already been diagnosed with coronary heart disease and has GTN (glyceryl trinitrate) spray or tablets, develops the above symptoms

(a)   (b)

Figure 5.1 (a) Glyceryl trinitrate spray and (b) tablets.

in the dental practice: often this will be angina that can be managed with rest and GTN, but it could be a myocardial infarction (heart attack) (British Heart Foundation, 2009). The patient should be managed as follows (British Heart Foundation, 2009):

- Ask the patient to stop what he is doing or sit down and rest.

- Ask the patient to take his GTN spray or tablets (Figure 5.1) as prescribed by his general practitioner. It is recommended that the dental practice should stock GTN, in case the patient doesn't have his own GTN with him (Resuscitation Council (UK), 2006).

- If the pain has not eased within a few minutes, ask the patient to take a second dose.

- If, after the repeated dose, the pain does not ease within a few minutes, call 999 for an ambulance immediately. In addition, if the patient is not allergic to aspirin, administer 300 mg (ask him to chew it); this is administered for its anti-platelet effect (British Medical Association & Royal Pharmaceutical Society, 2008).

- Even if the symptoms do not match the ones above but it is suspected that the patient is having a myocardial infarction, call 999 for an ambulance immediately.

NB, patients with known angina are usually asked to have their GTN spray easily accessible when attending for dental treatment.

MANAGEMENT OF MYOCARDIAL INFARCTION

Every 6 minutes someone dies from a heart attack
Every 11 minutes a man dies from a heart attack
Every 13 minutes a woman dies from a heart attack
(British Heart Foundation, 2009)

In the UK alone, over 146,000 people each year have a myocardial infarction (British Heart Foundation, 2009). Myocardial infarction is the leading cause of death in the UK (Wyatt *et al.*, 2006), accounting for 90,000 deaths each year (British Heart Foundation, 2009).

Of sudden cardiac deaths 50% occur within the first hour of onset, and 75% within three hours of onset, of an acute myocardial infarction (Laird *et al.*, 2004). The most common cause of death is ventricular fibrillation (Jevon, 2009).

The risk of this, together with the life-saving benefits of coronary reperfusion therapy (see below), reinforces the importance of ensuring that the dental practice dials 999 for an ambulance if a patient is suspected of having an myocardial infarction (Jevon, 2006): approximately 1.4 million people over the age of 35 years living in the UK have survived a heart attack (British Heart Foundation, 2009).

There are two practical methods of coronary reperfusion therapy: thrombolytic drug therapy and percutaneous transluminal coronary angioplasty (PTCA) (Jevon, 2006). The benefits of thrombolytic therapy in the management of an acute myocardial infarction are well documented: a recent overview of all randomised trials showed a short-term reduction in mortality of 24% (Jevon, 2009). The effect on mortality has been shown to continue for up to 10 years (GISSI, 1998).

Aspirin 300 mg (Figure 5.2) is a key treatment therapy, particularly in the pre-hospital situation (British Heart Foundation, 2009), as it reduces the incidence of coronary reocclusion following thrombolytic therapy, reducing the incidence of cardiac death. It should be administered as soon as possible as long as the patient is not allergic to it or has an active peptic ulcer (Wyatt *et al.*, 2005). If aspirin is chewed, it is absorbed more quickly than if it is swallowed, in the early stages of an acute myocardial infarction (Resuscitation Council UK, 2006).

Figure 5.2 Aspirin 300 mg.

Pathogenesis

A myocardial infarction is usually caused by the rupture of an atheromatous plaque in a coronary artery (Chesebro *et al.*, 1997). Prior to rupture, the majority of these plaques are not haemodynamically significant (Ambrose & Fuster, 1997). However, once the plaque ruptures the following events are triggered:

- Haemorrhage into the plaque. This causes it to expand and restrict the lumen of the coronary artery;
- Contraction of the smooth muscle in the artery wall, which will further restrict the lumen;
- Thrombus formation on the surface of the ruptured plaque (platelet adhesion) leading to total obstruction of the coronary lumen (Jevon, 2006).

Signs and symptoms

Common or typical symptoms include:

- Central chest pain;
- The pain can spread to the arms, neck or jaw;
- Feeling sick or sweaty as well as having central chest pain;
- Feeling short of breath as well as having central chest pain.

Symptoms vary and some people may feel any of the following:

- A dull pain, ache, or 'heavy' feeling in the chest;
- A mild discomfort in the chest making the patient feel generally unwell;
- The pain in the chest can spread to the back or stomach;
- A chest pain that feels like a bad episode of indigestion;
- Feeling a bit light-headed or dizzy as well as having chest pain.
  (British Heart Foundation, 2009).

> Sometimes the history can be unhelpful, e.g. a myocardial infarction may develop without any significant chest pain. Sometimes it is difficult to distinguish between cardiac and indigestion pains

CARDIAC DISORDERS

Figure 5.3 Sit the patient down (lie him flat if in shock).

Treatment

- If the patient displays the above symptoms and has not been diagnosed with heart disease, call 999 immediately (British Heart Foundation, 2009).

- Help the patient to adopt a relaxed position, which reduces the myocardial workload: he will usually prefer to sit with his head and shoulders supported and his knees bent (Resuscitation Council (UK), 2006; British Heart Foundation, 2003) (Figure 5.3). Note: a supine position can sometimes provoke or worsen the pain. However, particularly if the patient is in shock, he may benefit from lying down (Resuscitation Council (UK), 2006).

- Reassure the patient and encourage him to rest.

- Ideally, administer supplementary oxygen (British Medical Association & Royal Pharmaceutical Society, 2008).

- Ask the patient if he is allergic to aspirin. If he is not, administer aspirin 300 mg: ask him to chew it. It is administered for its anti-platelet effect (British Medical Association & Royal Pharmaceutical Society, 2008). Remember to send a note with the patient to hospital saying that aspirin has been administered (British Medical Association & Royal Pharmaceutical Society, 2008).

- If the patient has GTN spray or tablets, encourage him to use it as prescribed by his GP. It is recommended that the dental practice has GTN available in its emergency drug kit – this could be administered if necessary (Resuscitation Council (UK), 2006). Do warn the patient that a side effect of GTN is a headache.

- Closely monitor the patient; there is a risk of cardiopulmonary arrest.

Figure 5.4 British Heart Foundation's 'Doubt Kills' chest pain awareness campaign (2008).

There are many reasons why people delay calling 999 for an ambulance, e.g. uncertainty about the symptoms or not wishing to make a fuss (British Heart Foundation, 2009). The British Heart Foundation's *Doubt Kills* campaign in 2008 (Figure 5.4), stressed the importance of calling 999

MANAGEMENT OF PALPITATIONS

Palpitations is when the patient has a noticeable rapid, strong or irregular heartbeat (Soanes & Stevenson, 2006). Palpitations characteristically start and end abruptly.

Causes

Causes of palpitations include:

- ischaemic heart disease;

Figure 5.5 Example of a vagal manoeuvre: ask the patient to attempt to blow the plunger out of a syringe.

- drugs;
- tea or coffee;
- alcohol;
- stress (Jevon, 2006).

Treatment

- Sit the patient down and ask him if he has had palpitations previously.
- Reassure the patient.
- Try vagal stimulation: the most effective way of doing this is a Valsalva manoeuvre (the action of attempting to exhale with the nostrils or mouth or glottis closed; Soanes & Stevenson, 2006) in the supine position (Wyatt *et al.*, 2006); ask the patient to cough or hold his nose and blow as if to pop his ears (Keech, 2004); another option is to ask the patient to attempt to blow the plunger out of a syringe (Figure 5.5) (impossible to do, but a safe effective vagal manoeuvre).
- If the patient is symptomatic, e.g. breathless, light-headed or has chest pain, call 999 for an ambulance; if the patient is not symptomatic, but the palpitations do not settle, seek medical advice (Keech, 2004).

(source: Jevon, 2006)

MANAGEMENT OF SYNCOPE

Syncope (derived from the Greek word meaning 'to cut short') can be defined as a brief loss of consciousness caused by a fall in blood pressure (Soanes & Stevenson, 2006). The commonest cause of syncope is a vasovagal attack or simple faint (British Medical Association & Royal Pharmaceutical Society, 2008). The term *vasovagal* relates to or denotes a temporary fall in blood pressure with pallor, fainting, sweating and nausea caused by overactivity of the vagus nerve, particularly as a result of stress (Soanes & Stevenson, 2006). Vasovagal syncope is the commonest medical emergency encountered in the dental practice, accounting for approximately two-thirds of all emergencies (Müller *et al.*, 2008).

It is estimated that 30% of the population have experienced a fainting episode and many more have observed friends or colleagues have one (Benditt & Goldstein, 2002).

Causes

In the dental practice the most likely cause of a syncope episode is stress. Other possible causes include:

- warm environment;
- prolonged standing;
- sudden fright;
- visual stimulus, e.g. sight of blood, sight of a needle;
- the bill!

Signs and symptoms

Signs and symptoms that may be evident include:

- sense of feeling unwell;
- light-headedness or dizziness;
- nausea and vomiting;
- sudden tiredness;
- yawning;

- blurred or tunnel vision;

- pallor;

- sudden collapse (Wyatt *et al.*, 2006).

If the patient remains in an upright position, seizure-type twitching may occur (convulsive syncope) (Wyatt *et al.*, 2006).

Treatment

- If the patient feels faint, advise him to lie down; put the dental chair in a horizontal position. Raising the bottom end of the chair can be helpful.

- If the patient starts to collapse, if possible support him to the floor, taking care not to sustain an injury while doing so.

- Call out for help.

- Assess ABC to rule out cardiopulmonary arrest; as soon as the patient is horizontal he will usually start to regain consciousness.

- If the patient has collapsed on the floor, kneel down and raise the his legs above the level of his heart (Figure 5.6).

- Ensure a supply of fresh air, e.g. loosen any light clothing around the neck and chest, open a nearby window or door and ask colleagues not to crowd around the patient.

- Reassure the patient.

Figure 5.6 Dealing with a faint: lie the patient flat and raise the legs.

- Check for any injuries; if the patient collapses during a faint, injuries e.g. bone fractures or a head injury could be sustained, particularly in the elderly (Benditt & Goldstein, 2002).

- Note the duration of the syncope episode; if a simple faint, the patient will quickly recover, usually within 60 seconds (Benditt & Goldstein, 2002).

- Once the patient regains consciousness, offer a drink e.g. sugar in water or a cup of sweet tea (British Medical Association & Royal Pharmaceutical Society, 2008).

- If the patient takes time to recover, place him in the recovery position. Assess the patient following the ABCDE approach. It may be necessary to call 999 for an ambulance.

Other considerations

- Always distinguish between an innocent 'simple faint' and a collapse due to a more sinister reason, e.g. a seizure or a cardiac event (Wyatt *et al.*, 2006). Cyanosis, tongue biting, saliva frothing at the mouth or incontinence suggest a generalised seizure (Wyatt *et al.*, 2006).

- Note any neurological signs during the episode (Wyatt *et al.*, 2006).

- Advise the patient to recognise and avoid situations that could cause him to faint (Benditt & Goldstein, 2002).

CONCLUSION

Coronary heart disease is the leading cause of death in the UK. Chest pain, a characteristic symptom of coronary heart disease, is the commonest reason for alerting the emergency services. In this chapter, the management of angina and myocardial infarction have been discussed in detail. The management of palpitations and syncope have also been outlined.

REFERENCES

Ambrose J, Fuster V (1997) Can we predict future acute coronary events in patients with stable coronary artery disease? (editorial; comment). *JAMA*; 277:343–344.
Benditt D, Goldstein M (2002) Fainting. *Circulation*; 106:1048–1050.
British Heart Foundation (2009) www.bhf.org.uk (accessed 10/02/09).
British Medical Association & Royal Pharmaceutical Society of Great Britain (2008) *British National Formulary 56*. BMJ Publishing, London.

Chesebro J, Rauch U, Fuster V, Badimon J (1997) Pathogenesis of thrombosis in coronary artery disease. *Haemostasis*; 27(suppl 1):12–18.

GISSI (1998) Ten-year follow-up of the first megatrial testing thrombolytic therapy in patients with acute myocardial infarction: results of the GISSI study. *Circulation*; 98:2659–2665.

Jevon P (2006) *Emergency Care & First Aid for Nurses*. Elsevier, Oxford.

Jevon P (2009) *Advanced Cardiac Life Support*, 2nd edn. Wiley-Blackwell, Oxford.

Keech P (2004) *Practical Guide to First Aid*. Lorenz Books, London.

Laird C, Driscoll P, Wardrope J (2004) The ABC of community emergency care. 3 Chest pain. *Emergency Medicine Journal*; 21;226–232.

Müller M, Hänsel M, Stehr S *et al.* (2008) A state-wide survey of medical emergency management in dental practices: incidence of emergencies and training experience. *Emergency Medicine Journal*; 25; 296–300.

Resuscitation Council (UK) (2006) *Medical emergencies and resuscitation standards for clinical practice and training for dental practitioners and dental care professionals in general dental practice*. Resuscitation Council (UK), London.

Soanes C, Stevenson A (2006) *Oxford Dictionary of English*, 2nd edn. Oxford University Press, Oxford.

Wyatt J, Illingworth R, Graham C *et al.* (2006) *Oxford Handbook of Emergency Medicine*, 3rd edn. Oxford University Press, Oxford.

CARDIAC DISORDERS

Chapter 6

Neurological disorders

INTRODUCTION

Neurological disorders account for approximately 20% of admissions to general hospitals in the UK, an increasing proportion of which are emergencies (Sharief & Anand, 1997). Neurological disorders can be life threatening; altered consciousness level can lead to a compromised airway and compromised breathing. Neurological disorders in the dental practice require prompt effective treatment, together with close monitoring of ABCDE to detect deterioration.

The aim of this chapter is to understand the management of neurological disorders.

LEARNING OUTCOMES

At the end of this chapter the reader will be able to:

- Discuss the management of a generalised tonic-clonic seizure
- Discuss the management of a stroke
- Discuss the management of altered level of consciousness
- Describe the procedure for placing a patient in the recovery position

MANAGEMENT OF A GENERALISED TONIC-CLONIC SEIZURE

A seizure is caused by a sudden burst of electrical activity in all or part of the brain (Epilepsy Action, 2009). Approximately 2–10% of the population will experience a seizure at some time in their life (National Institute for Clinical Excellence, 2002). There are over 40 different types of seizure, a person may have more than one type and recurrent seizures are defined as epilepsy (Epilepsy Action, 2009). In this section the management of a patient having a generalised tonic-clonic seizure, sometimes called a grand mal fit, will be discussed. In the dental practice, these seizures account for approximately 7% of all medical emergencies encountered in the dental surgery (Müller *et al.*, 2008).

Sudden unexpected death in epilepsy accounts for approximately 500 deaths each year (National Institute for Clinical Excellence, 2002). Status epilepticus, a potentially life-threatening medical emergency, is associated with significant morbidity and mortality if not treated promptly (National Institute for Clinical Excellence, 2002). Injuries that can be sustained include fractures, burns, dislocations, concussion and intracerebral haemorrhage (American Heart Association, 2005). Dental injuries are quite common (Buck *et al.*, 1997). Maintaining the patient's safety during a seizure is a priority.

Signs and symptoms

Typical characteristics of a generalised tonic-clonic seizure (Jevon, 2006; Turner, 2007; Epilepsy Action, 2009; St John Ambulance *et al.*, 2006) include:

- Sudden loss of consciousness (can be preceded by crying out) and collapse to the ground;
- Rigidity (tonic phase) – lasting for approximately 10 seconds, the body is stiff, the elbows are flexed and the legs are extended;
- Breathing stops; central cyanosis particularly noticeable around the mouth
- Clenching of the jaw – saliva may accumulate at the mouth, which could be blood-stained if the casualty has bitten his tongue or lip;
- Convulsive movements (clonic phase) – lasting for 1–2 minutes, there is violent generalised rhythmical shaking;
- Incontinence;
- Variable period of unconsciousness following the event. The casualty may feel very tired and may fall into a deep sleep; he could be dazed, confused, disorientated, frightened and may have slurred, incomprehensible speech.

Causes

Causes of a generalised tonic-clonic seizure include:

- epilepsy (most common cause);
- head injury;
- certain poisons, e.g. alcohol, ecstasy;
- alcohol withdrawal;

NEUROLOGICAL DISORDERS

- cerebral hypoxia;
- cerebral hypoglycaemia (Jevon, 2006).

Treatment

- If necessary, call 999 for an ambulance (see below).
- Ensure that it is safe to approach the patient.
- Protect the patient from injury. Ensure the space around him is clear and remove any objects that are potentially dangerous objects.
- Loosen any clothing around the patient's neck.
- Cushion the patient's head, e.g. place something soft such as a pillow, jumper or jacket under his head. Alternatively, place the palms of your hands behind his head and support it to prevent injury.
- Note the time in order to check how long the seizure lasts.
- Once the seizure has stopped check airway, breathing and circulation; if the patient is breathing place him into the recovery position (if the patient is not breathing, start resuscitation).
- Wipe away any saliva; suction may be necessary.
- Check to see whether the patient has sustained any injuries.
- Calmly reassure the patient.
- Stay with the patient until he has made a complete recovery.
- Administer oxygen to support breathing if necessary.
- Consider medication if the convulsive (jerking) movements are prolonged (5 minutes or longer) or if the seizures are repeated rapidly; midazolam10 mg (buccal liquid or injection) administered by the buccal route (unlicensed use) is recommended (Figure 6.1) (British Medical Association & Royal Pharmaceutical Society, 2008).

(St John Ambulance *et al.*, 2006; Jevon & Morgan, 2007; Epilepsy Action, 2009; National Society for Epilepsy, 2009)

When to call 999 for an ambulance

Call 999 for an ambulance if:

- it is the patient's first seizure; or
- the seizure continues for longer than 5 minutes; or

NEUROLOGICAL DISORDERS

- one tonic-clonic seizure follows another without the casualty regaining consciousness between seizures (status epilepticus); or

- the patient incurs an injury during the seizure; or

- the patient requires urgent medical attention; or

1 Open the bottle, check the plunger of the oral dosing applicator is pressed to the bottom and firmly insert the oral dosing applicator into the bung on top of the bottle.

2 Holding the bottle, tip it upside down and slowly pull back on the oral dosing applicator plunger (to release the air) and return. Then pull back on the oral dosing applicator plunger until you have withdrawn the amount prescribed. Put the lid back on the bottle immediately to prevent the medicine evaporating.

3 If the child/young person/adult has no head support on a chair, support the head by standing behind them, holding the chin. Be careful not to press on the throat.

4 If the child/young person/adult is lying on the floor or if a chair has a head support in place, hold the chin to keep the head steady.

5 Open the mouth gently by holding the chin, apply downward pressure on the lower lip and wipe away any excess saliva (no need to part the teeth).

Figure 6.1 Buccal administration of midazolam. Reproduced with permission from Special Products Ltd.

Place the nozzle of the oral dosing applicator between the lower gum and the cheek on one side of the mouth (the buccal cavity). Slowly give half the prescribed amount of Midazolam into the mouth, remove the oral dosing applicator, close the lips together and rub the cheek on the outside. Repeat this on the other side of the mouth to give the remaining dose.

Do not give the medicine too quickly, as this may cause the child/young person/adult to choke or swallow it. If a small amount is swallowed it is not a problem.

Place the child/young person/adult in the recovery position, if appropriate.

Figure 6.1 (*Continued*)

- if there is difficulty monitoring the patient; or
- if there is a high risk of recurrence (Resuscitation Council (UK), 2006; Epilepsy Action, 2009; National Society of Epilepsy, 2009).

Action not recommended during a seizure

During a seizure it is recommended not to:

- Restrain the patient;
- Insert anything in the patient's mouth;
- Move the patient unless he is in danger;
- Give the patient anything to eat or drink until he has fully recovered;
- Attempt to arouse the patient.
  (Epilepsy Action, 2009).

Observations during a seizure

'A clear history from the casualty and an eyewitness to the attack give the most important diagnostic information, and should be the mainstay of diagnosis'

(Scottish Intercollegiate Guidelines Network, 2003). The following observations during a seizure will assist in its diagnosis and classification:

- Where was the patient and what was he doing prior to the seizure?
- Any mood change, e.g. excitement, anger or anxiety?
- Unusual sensations, e.g. odd smell or taste?
- Any prior warning?
- Loss of consciousness or confusion?
- Any colour change, e.g. pallor, cyanosis? If so where, e.g. face, lips, hand?
- Altered respiratory pattern, e.g. dyspnoea, noising respirations?
- Which part of the body affected by seizure?
- Incontinence?
- Tongue biting?
- Did the patient do anything unusual, e.g. mumble, wander about or fumble with his clothing?
- How long did the seizure last?
- How was the patient following the seizure? Did the patient need to sleep and, if so, for how long?
- How long before the patient can perform normal activities again?. (National Society of Epilepsy, 2009).

NEUROLOGICAL DISORDERS

MANAGEMENT OF STROKE

A stroke can be defined as a focal or global neurological deficit with symptoms lasting > 24 hours (Wyatt *et al.*, 2006). A stroke is a medical emergency; each year 150,000 people in the UK have a stroke, most of whom are over 65 years of age (Stroke Association, 2009). Stroke is the third biggest cause of death and the single most common cause of disability in the UK (Stroke Association, 2009). A patient suffering a stroke requires immediate treatment, which is directed towards sustaining life and preventing further brain damage (Jevon, 2006).

A transient ischaemic attack (TIA), sometimes called a mini-stroke, is when the brain's blood supply is interrupted for a brief time; although the symptoms are similar to a stroke they are only temporary, lasting minutes or hours but disappearing completely within 24 hours (Stroke Association, 2009). A transient ischaemic attack could lead to a major stroke: the patient should be reviewed by his GP as soon as possible and referred to a specialist stroke service within 7 days (Stroke Association, 2009).

Pathogenesis

A stroke is caused by either cerebral infarction or cerebral haemorrhage:

- *Cerebral infarction (80%)*: due to thrombosis, cerebral embolism (e.g. from atrial fibrillation or valve disease/replacement) or very occasionally an episode of hypoperfusion;

- *Cererbral haemorrhage (20%)*: associated with hypertension, subarachnoid haemorrhage and bleeding disorders.
  (Wyatt *et al.*, 2006).

Symptoms

The symptoms will depend on the type of stroke, the area affected and the extent of the stroke. Symptoms may include:

- sudden weakness or numbness of the face, arm or leg on one side of the body;

- sudden severe unexplained headache;

- sudden loss or blurring of vision, in one or both eyes;

- sudden difficulty in speaking or understanding spoken language;

- sudden confusion;

- loss of balance – dizziness, unsteadiness or a sudden fall, particularly with any of the above signs.
  (Stroke Association, 2009).

Recognition of a stroke: FAST

The Stroke Association (2009) recommends following the FAST (Figure 6.2) approach when assessing whether a patient has had a stroke:

- *Facial weakness*: can the patient smile? Has her mouth or an eye drooped?

- *Arm weakness*: can the patient raise both arms?

- *Speech problems*: can the patient speak clearly and understand what is being said to him?

- *Test all three symptoms.*

Figure 6.2 The Stroke Association's FAST guidelines for assessing a patient with a suspected stroke. Reproduced with kind permission of The Stroke Association.

These simple checks can help to ascertain whether the patient has had a stroke or not.

Treatment

- Assess the patient following the ABCDE approach described in chapter 3. Also assess the patient following the FAST approach (see above); if a stroke is suspected call 999 for an ambulance (Stroke Association, 2009).

- Ensure the patient has a clear airway. Following a stroke the airway can become compromised by the tongue and/or secretions in the mouth. Ensure the patient's airway remains patent: aspiration of gastric contents or secretions is a serious complication of a stroke, which is associated with considerable morbidity and mortality (American Heart Association, 2005).

- If the patient is unconscious (but breathing), place him in the recovery position; inserting an oropharyngeal airway may be helpful.

- If the patient is conscious, ensure his head and shoulders are supported in a slightly raised position, thus helping to protect the airway; tilting the head towards the affected side allows secretions to drain out; wipe the mouth with a flannel or similar (St John Ambulance *et al.*, 2006). It may be necessary to suction the mouth.

- Regularly monitor the patient's airway and do not give him anything to eat or drink (Wyatt *et al.*, 2006).

- Administer high flow oxygen using a non-rebreathe mask (Figure 3.1). If available, establish oxygen saturation monitoring using a pulse oximeter. Closely monitor the patient's breathing as ventilatory support may be required.

- Closely monitor the patient's vital signs.

- Closely monitor the patient's level of consciousness, using the AVPU scale.

- Reassure the patient. Once the patient regains consciousness the patient may be disorientated and may have a headache requiring analgesia.

MANAGEMENT OF ALTERED LEVEL OF CONSCIOUSNESS

The patient's level of consciousness has been described as the degree of his arousal and awareness (Geraghty, 2005). It is dependent upon the interaction of the ascending reticular activating system situated in the brainstem and the cerebral hemispheres (Jevon & Morgan, 2007). Any disruption in this communication process will result in altered consciousness (Bassett & Makin, 2000). The manifestation of altered consciousness implies an underlying brain dysfunction (Geraghty, 2005).

The term 'unconsciousness' can be defined as not awake, not aware of and not responding to one's environment (Soanes & Stevenson, 2006).

Causes

Causes of altered level of consciousness include:

- metabolic disturbances, e.g. hypoglycaemia, hypothyroidism;

- trauma, e.g. head injury;

- stroke;

- infection, e.g. meningitis;

- drugs, e.g. opiates, midazolam;

- alcohol.
  (Jevon, 2006).

Investigations

While awaiting the arrival of an ambulance, it would help to try to establish the possible cause of the unconsciousness, e.g. if able, check the patient's blood sugar for the presence of hypoglycaemia.

Treatment

If the patient appears to be unconscious and lifeless, follow the resuscitation protocols described in chapter 9 and start cardiopulmonary resuscitation immediately if required

Review ABCDE

- Assess the patient following the ABCDE approach described in chapter 3. As a compromised airway, inadequate breathing or inadequate circulation can lead to altered conscious level, attention to these is a priority (Wyatt et al., 2006).

- If necessary, call 999 for an ambulance.

- Ensure the patient has a clear airway. The airway can become compromised by the tongue and/or secretions, vomit, etc. in the mouth. If the patient is unconscious (but breathing), place in the recovery position (see below) and consider inserting an oropharyngeal airway (see pages 133–6). Regular oral suction may be required. If the patient has dentures, these are usually only removed if they are loose or ill-fitting.

- Regularly monitor the patient's airway (Wyatt et al., 2006).

- If necessary administer oxygen (Figure 3.1). If available, establish oxygen saturation monitoring using a pulse oximeter. Closely monitor the patient's respiratory rate as ventilatory support may be required.

- Closely monitor the patient's level of consciousness, using the AVPU scale, and undertake regular assessment of the pupils.

- If able, perform blood glucose measurement. Treat confirmed or suspected hypoglycaemia.

- Check the patient's medication history for recent administration of a mediation that may cause unconsciousness, e.g. an opiate.

PROCEDURE FOR PLACING A PATIENT IN THE RECOVERY POSITION

In an unconscious patient the airway is at risk. Regurgitated gastric contents, debris in the mouth or upper airway, loose dentures or mechanical obstruction arising from structures in the mouth, e.g. the tongue and epiglottis, can all compromise the airway (Quinn, 1998).

The recovery position is designed to maintain a patent airway and reduce the risk of airway obstruction and aspiration (American Heart Association, 2005). It is recommended in an unconscious patient who is breathing normally and has an effective circulation (American Heart Association, 2005).

Indications

The recovery position is advocated for most unconscious patients. In the situation following cardiac arrest, if the patient is breathing spontaneously and

NEUROLOGICAL DISORDERS

does not require any further resuscitation, then appropriate positioning of the patient using the recommended recovery position promotes the maintenance of a clear airway and helps prevent vomit or secretions from obstructing the airway and potentially causing aspiration.

The recovery position is also recommended in many other situations where the patient's conscious level is compromised, e.g. following a major seizure (Hayes, 2004; Bingham, 2004) and during a hypoglycaemic coma (Diebel, 1999).

Right or left lateral

Historically the left lateral position has been advocated for the recovery position (Eastwick-Field, 1996). However, there appears to be no cardiac autonomic tone advantages to be gained by placing a person in the recovery position on one side compared with the other (Ryan et al., 2003). Although either side can be used, in practical terms the environment can dictate which side is used, e.g. if the patient has collapsed next to a wall, he will have to be rolled away from it. In the dental chair, it would be sensible to position the patient so that he is facing the suction apparatus.

Variations

There are several different variations of the recovery position, each with its own advantages (Resuscitation Council (UK), 2005). However, no single technique is perfect for all patients (Turner et al., 1998; Handley, 1993). The position used should be stable, near a true lateral position with the head dependent and no pressure applied to the chest which could impair breathing (American Heart Association, 2005).

Procedure – patient on the floor

- Check the environment and decide which is the best side to roll the patient. Remove any obstacles if necessary.

- If necessary, remove the patient's spectacles and place them in a safe place. Some authorities also recommend checking in the patient's pockets and removing any sharp instruments, e.g. keys. If doing this proceed with extreme caution.

- Loosen any clothing around the neck.

- Kneel beside the patient. To minimise the risk of self-injury, adopt a stable base with the knees a shoulder-width apart, avoid twisting the back

Figure 6.3 The recovery position: hold the back of the hand against the patient's cheek.

and keep the spine in a neutral position (Resuscitation Council (UK), 2001).

- Ensure that both of the patient's legs are straight.

- Position the arm nearest to the dental practitioner perpendicular to the patient's body with the elbow bent and the hand palm uppermost.

- Grasp the far arm and bring it across the patient's chest and hold the back of the hand against the patient's cheek (Figure 6.3).

- Using the free hand, grasp the far leg just above the knee and pull it up, taking care to keep the patient's foot on the ground (Figure 6.4).

- While holding the patient's hand against his cheek, pull on the far leg to roll the patient towards you onto his side (Figure 6.5).

- Tilt the patient's head back to ensure that the airway remains open (Figure 6.6).

- If necessary, adjust the hand under the patient's cheek to maintain the head tilted.

- Monitor the patient's vital signs.

(Resuscitation Council (UK), 2005)

NEUROLOGICAL DISORDERS

Figure 6.4 The recovery position: grasp the far leg just above the knee and pull it up.

Figure 6.5 The recovery position: whilst holding the patient's hand against his cheek, pull on the far leg to roll the patient towards you onto his side.

Figure 6.6 The recovery position: tilt the patient's head back to ensure that the airway remains open.

Procedure – patient in the dental chair

Due to limited space, it is very difficult to follow the above procedure when trying to place a patient with altered consciousness in the chair in the recovery position. It will usually be necessary to adapt the procedure. *Note:* there is the potential hazard of the patient rolling off the chair onto the floor. Great care should be taken when attempting to place the patient in the lateral position in the dental chair.

Safer handling

Guidelines from the Resuscitation Council (UK) (2001) on safer handling during resuscitation should be observed to reduce the risk of self-injury:

- Assess the situation;
- Adopt a position close to and directly facing the patient;
- Avoid twisting the back;
- Keep the spine in a neutral position;
- Face the patient straight on.

Complications

Even if the patient is in the recovery position, airway, breathing and circulation can still become compromised. Closely monitor the patient's vital signs, particularly breathing (Resuscitation Council (UK), 2005).

It has been reported that when the lower arm is placed in front, compression of vessels and nerves in the dependent limb can occur (Fulstow & Smith, 1993;

NEUROLOGICAL DISORDERS

Turner *et al.*, 1998). Therefore monitor for signs of impaired blood flow in the lowermost arm (Rathgeber *et al.*, 1996) and ensure that the duration for which there is pressure on this arm is kept to a minimum (Resuscitation Council (UK), 2005). If the patient needs to remain in the recovery position for longer than 30 minutes, turn him to the opposite side to relieve pressure on the forearm (Resuscitation Council (UK), 2005).

SPINAL INJURY

The author acknowledges that the risk of encountering a spinal injury in the dental practice is extremely rare. However, for completeness, it was considered important to consider it here.

If the patient has a known or suspected spinal injury, he should only be moved if an open airway cannot otherwise be maintained. Ideally the patient should be kept still in the position he is found, while awaiting the arrival of the emergency services. However if it is necessary to move the patient, e.g. because of compromised airway, the patient should ideally be carefully log-rolled, with the head and neck kept as still as possible and in alignment. Extension of the lower arm above the head together with bending both legs, while rolling the head onto the arm, may be feasible (American Heart Association, 2005).

CONCLUSION

Neurological disorders can be life threatening and can occur in the dental practice. An altered consciousness level can lead to a compromised airway and compromised breathing which, if untreated, may lead to cardiopulmonary arrest. The patient should be assessed following the ABCDE approach. In this chapter the management of seizures, stroke and altered level of consciousness have been discussed. In addition, the recovery position, which is often indicated in a patient with a neurological disorder, has been described.

REFERENCES

American Heart Association (2005) 2005 American Heart Association Guidelines for Cardiopulmonary Resuscitation and Emergency cardiovascular care. *Circulation*; 112:24 suppl.

Bassett C, Makin L (eds) (2000) *Caring for the Seriously Ill Patient*. Arnold, London.

Bingham E (2004) Epilepsy: diagnosis and support for people with epilepsy. *Practice Nursing*; 15(2):64–70.

British Medical Association & Royal Pharmaceutical Society of Great Britain (2008) *British National Formulary 56*. BMJ Publishing, London.

Buck D, Baker G, Jacoby A *et al.* (1997) Patients' experiences of injury as a result of epilepsy. *Epilepsia*; 38(4):439–444.

NEUROLOGICAL DISORDERS

Diebel G (1999) The management of hypoglycaemia in type 1 and type 2 diabetes. *British Journal of Community Nursing*; 4(9):454–460.

Eastwick-Field P (1996) Resuscitation: basic life support. *Nursing Standard*; 10(34):49–56.

Epilepsy Action (2009) Epilepsy Information: First Aid For Seizures (www .epilespy.org.uk).

Fulstow R, Smith G (1993) The new recovery position, a cautionary tale. *Resuscitation*; 26:89–91.

Geraghty M (2005) Nursing the unconscious patient. *Nursing Standard*; 20(1):54–64.

Handley A (1993) Recovery position. *Resuscitation*; 26:93–95.

Hayes C (2004) Clinical skills: practical guide for managing adults with epilepsy. *British Journal of Nursing*; 13(7):380–387.

Jevon P (2006) *Emergency Care & First Aid for Nurses*. Elsevier, Oxford.

Jevon P, Morgan A (2007) First aid part 2 – treatment of a generalised tonic-clonic seizure. *Nursing Times*; 103(51):24–25.

Müller M, Hänsel M, Stehr S *et al.* (2008) A state-wide survey of medical emergency management in dental practices: incidence of emergencies and training experience. *Emergency Medicine Journal*; 25:296–300.

National Institute for Clinical Excellence (2002) Press Release: 2002/026 NICE launches National Clinical audit of epilepsy-related death (www.nice.org.uk).

National Society for Epilepsy (2009) *Epilepsy: what to do when someone has a seizure*. National Society for Epilepsy, Chalfont St Peter, Bucks.

Quinn T (1998) Cardiopulmonary resuscitation: new European guidelines. *British Journal of Nursing*; 7(18):1070–1077.

Rathgeber J, Panzer W, Gunther U *et al.* (1996) influence of different types of recovery positions on perfusion indices of the forearm. *Resuscitation*; 32:13–17.

Resuscitation Council UK (2001) *Guidance for Safer Handling during Resuscitation in Hospitals*. Resuscitation Council (UK), London.

Resuscitation Council (UK) (2005) *Guidelines 2005*. Resuscitation Council (UK), London

Resuscitation Council UK (2006) *Medical emergencies and resuscitation standards for clinical practice and training for dental practitioners and dental care professionals in general dental practice*. Resuscitation Council (UK), London.

Ryan A, Larsen P, Galletly D (2003) Comparison of heart rate variability in supine, and left and right lateral positions. *Anaesthesia*; 58(5):432–436.

Sharief M, Anand P (1997) Neurological emergencies. In Skinner D et al. (eds) *Cambridge Textbook of Accident & Emergency Medicine*. Cambridge University Press, Cambridge.

St John Ambulance, St Andrew's Ambulance, British Red Cross (2006) *First Aid Manual*, 9th edn. Dorling Kindersley, London.

Scottish Intercollegiate Guidelines Network (2003) *Diagnosis and management of epilepsy in adults*. SIGN, Edinburgh.

Soanes C, Stevenson A (2006) *Oxford Dictionary of English*, 2nd edn. Oxford University Press, Oxford.

The Stroke Association (2009) www.stroke.org.uk (accessed 12/02/2009).

Turner C (2007) *Neurology*, 2nd edn. Mosby, London.

Turner S, Turner I, Chapman D *et al.* (1998) A comparative study of the 1992 and 1997 recovery positions for use in the UK. *Resuscitation*; 39:153–160.

Wyatt J, Illingworth R, Graham C *et al.* (2006) *Oxford Handbook of Emergency Medicine*, 3rd edn. Oxford University Press, Oxford.

Chapter 7

Endocrine disorders

INTRODUCTION

Endocrine disorders account for approximately 1.5% of all hospital emergency admissions in England; the majority are related to diabetes (Kearney & Dang, 2007). In the dental practice, hypoglycaemia is by far the most likely endocrine disorder to be encountered. Adrenal insufficiency may also occur.

The aim of this chapter is to understand the management of endocrine disorders.

LEARNING OUTCOMES

At the end of this chapter the reader will be able to:

- Discuss the management of hypoglycaemia
- Describe the procedure for blood glucose measurement using a glucometer
- Discuss the management of adrenal insufficiency

MANAGEMENT OF HYPOGLYCAEMIA

Hypoglycaemia is normally defined as a blood glucose level < 3 mmols/l (Resuscitation Council (UK), 2006) and is usually associated with diabetes (particularly patients taking insulin). When attending for dental treatment, diabetic patients should eat as normal and should take their medication, e.g. insulin or oral hypoglycaemic agent, as prescribed (Resuscitation Council (UK), 2006; British Medical Association & Royal Pharmaceutical Society, 2008). If a meal is missed, then hypoglycaemia can occur (British Medical Association & Royal Pharmaceutical Society, 2008).

Incidence

The exact incidence of hypoglycaemic episodes in the general population is unknown, as most are treated successfully at home and some, particularly those occurring at night, may not even be recognised. On average there are over 90,000 calls to the emergency services each year for hypoglycaemia (Sampson et al., 2006). In 2004/5 there were 8000 admissions to hospital in England due to hypoglycaemia (Kearney & Dang, 2007).

Hypoglycaemia accounts for approximately 22% of medical emergencies encountered in the dental surgery (Müller et al., 2008). Diabetic patients treated with insulin are most likely to become hypoglycaemic while attending for dental treatment (Resuscitation Council (UK), 2006).

Risks

The risks associated with hypoglycaemia are small, though altered level of consciousness can always lead to airway compromise. However, hypoglycaemia can cause an acute cerebral injury, leading to hemiplegia (Shirayama et al., 2004); a prolonged severe hypoglycaemic episode can even cause moderate to severe neuropsychological impairments (Kubiak et al., 2004).

Causes of hypoglycaemia

Common causes of hypoglycaemia include:

- too much insulin;
- delayed or missed meal or snack;
- insufficient food, especially carbohydrate;
- unplanned or strenuous exercise;
- alcohol consumption without food;
- idiopathic.
  (Diabetes UK, 2009).

  Medical causes of hypoglycaemia include:

- liver failure;
- Addison's disease;
- pituitary insufficiency.
  (Wyatt et al., 2006).

ENDOCRINE DISORDERS

Nearly all hypoglycaemic episodes occur in patients who are prescribed insulin treatment, though episodes may rarely occur in patients prescribed sulphonylurea drugs (Shorr *et al.*, 1997); these drugs, e.g. glibenclamide, augment insulin production (British Medical Association & Royal Pharmaceutical Society, 2008).

Consumption of alcohol can lead to hypoglycaemia several hours later; in addition the effects of alcohol can mask the symptoms of hypoglycaemia.

Clinical features

The clinical features of hypoglycaemia vary from person to person, though they are often constant for an individual (Diabetes UK, 2009). Individuals may recognise different symptoms and these may change as the duration of diabetes increases (McLaren & Somerville, 1988).

Clinical features of hypoglycaemia can be classified as either autonomic (usually present first when the blood glucose is 3.3–3.6 mmol/l) or related to neuroglycopenia (usually present when the blood glucose is < 2.6 mmol/l):

- *Autonomic:* sweating, hunger, hot sensation, anxiety, nausea and vomiting;
- *Neuroglycopenia:* fatigue, visual disturbance, uncoordinated and altered behaviour, drowsiness, confusion and if untreated convulsions and coma (Kearney & Dang, 2007; British Medical Association & Royal Pharmaceutical Society, 2008; Diabetes UK, 2009).

Note: in patients with chronic hypergycaemia, the autonomic clinical features may be triggered at higher blood glucose levels (Boyle *et al.*, 1988).

The patient is usually aware that he is developing hypoglycaemia (Diabetes UK, 2009), though this may not always be the case. In addition, recurrent hypoglycaemic episodes can lead to diminished casualty awareness of impending hypoglycaemia (Watkins, 2003; Kearney & Dang, 2007). The dental practitioner should therefore always be alert to the clinical features of hypoglycaemia.

Diagnosis

Ideally blood glucose measurement should be undertaken in the dental practice. It is recommended that each dental practice has an automated blood glucose measurement device (Resuscitation Council (UK), 2006). The biomedical diagnosis of hypoglycaemia is a blood sugar < 3.0 mmol/litre (Resuscitation Council (UK), 2006). A suggested procedure for blood glucose measurement is described in described on pages 98–9.

Figure 7.1 Glucose 10 mg.

Treatment

- Assess the patient following the ABCDE approach described in chapter 3. Treatment will depend upon the patient's level of consciousness and degree of co-operation (Wyatt *et al.*, 2006; Resuscitation Council (UK), 2006).

- If the patient's consciousness level allows him to safely eat and drink, offer him the simplest available and quickly absorbed food or drink that contains carbohydrate, e.g. milk with added sugar, a glass of Lucozade or cola (not diet drinks), a glass of fruit juice, or three or more glucose tablets (Diabetes UK, 2009). Repeat this after 10–15 minutes if necessary (British Medical Association & Royal Pharmaceutical Society (2008). This can then be followed by long-acting carbohydrates, e.g. digestive biscuits (Kearney & Dang, 2007).

- GlucoGel (Figure 7.1; formerly known as Hypostop), a dextrose gel stocked in most dental surgeries, is rapidly absorbed via the buccal mucosa. Gluco-Gel or similar may be administered (British Medical Association & Royal Pharmaceutical Society, 2008; Kearney & Dang, 2007).

In more severe cases, where the patient's level of consciousness deteriorates:

- Ensure his airway is clear and maintained; place him in the lateral position. If he is unconscious consider inserting a basic airway device, e.g. oropharyngeal airway (see pages 133–6).

- Administer high flow oxygen using a non-rebreathe mask (see pages 37–9). If available, attach pulse oximetry to monitor oxygen saturation.

- Administer glucagon 1 mg (Figure 7.2) IM/SC (hormone produced by the A-cells of the islets in the pancreas); it increases the blood glucose level by mobilising glycogen stores in the liver (Watkins, 2003). The majority of people with type 1 diabetes lose their glucagon response to hypoglycaemia within five years of diagnosis (Bolli et al., 1983). The recommended dose for glucagon is 1 mg subcutaneously or intramuscularly (British Medical Association & Royal Pharmaceutical Society, 2008). The procedure for administering glucagon is described in Box 7.1.

Figure 7.2 Glucagon.

ENDOCRINE DISORDERS

- Monitor the patient's response and level of consciousness; 90% of patients will fully recover in 20 minutes (Wyatt *et al.*, 2006).

- If able, recheck the blood glucose after 10 minutes to ensure that it has improved (5 mmol/l or more), in conjunction with an improvement in the patient's level of consciousness and AVPU scale (Resuscitation Council (UK), 2006).

- Try to establish the possible cause of the hypoglycaemia. To prevent a repeat hypoglycaemic episode, offer the patient food that contains starchy carbo-hydrates (absorbed more slowly), e.g. a sandwich, fruit or biscuits and milk (Diabetes (UK), 2009).

- Educate the patient. Education is the key to preventing recurrent or severe hypoglycaemia. It may be necessary to advise the patient to make an appointment to go to see his GP or practice nurse for assessment and advice.

- Reassure the patient. Repeated episodes of hypoglycaemia may cause extreme emotional distress, even when the episodes are relatively mild (Chelliah & Mark, 2004).

- If it was necessary to administer glucagon to the patient, he may go home once fully recovered, but should be accompanied; he should not drive and his GP should be informed (Resuscitation Council (UK), 2006).

When to call 999 for an ambulance

For some patients with hypoglycaemia, it will definitely be necessary to call 999 for an ambulance, particularly if the cause is an oral anti-diabetic drug (British Medical Association & Royal Pharmaceutical Society, 2008).

Box 7.1   Procedure for administering glucagon. With kind permission from Novo Nordisk Ltd.

Using GlucaGen®HypoKit Step by Step Guide

Instructions for use

1. Remove the orange plastic cap of the GlucaGen bottle. Insert the needle through the rubber seal disk on the bottle. Inject all the liquid in the syringe into the bottle. The rubber seal can be stiff, but the needle is strong enough to puncture it.

2. Leave the syringe in place and gently shake the bottle until the powder is completely dissolved, and the solution is clear.

3. Make sure the plunger is totally down, then gently pull it out until all the solution is drawn up into the syringe.

4. Ensure that there is no air in the syringe, before the injection is given. Pinch up the skin and inject the needle into it, for example in the outer thigh. You cannot harm the person by giving this injection.

5. After the injection, when the person responds, give a sweet drink like juice or a soft drink, to keep blood glucose levels up. Follow this up as soon as possible with a meal or snack.

ENDOCRINE DISORDERS

ENDOCRINE DISORDERS

PROCEDURE FOR BLOOD GLUCOSE MEASUREMENT USING A GLUCOMETER

The procedure for blood glucose measurement involves obtaining a small sample of the patient's blood, usually from his fingertip, and applying it to a test strip inserted into an electronic meter (glucometer) (Figure 7.3). The result is expressed in millimoles per litre (mmol/l), i.e. it is a measurement of millimoles of glucose per litre of blood. It is recommended that a glucometer should be available in the dental practice (Resuscitation Council (UK), 2006).

Indications

In the dental practice, it would be helpful to undertake blood glucose measurement if hypoglycaemia (see pages 98–9) is suspected, or after a seizure (Resuscitation Council (UK), 2006).

Procedure

Described below is a typical procedure for blood glucose measurement using a glucometer device. It is important to follow the manufacturer's recommendations for the specific device being used in the dental practice.

- Explain the procedure to the patient.

- Assemble equipment: glucometer (ensure that a high/low test has been done as recommended by the manufacturer), finger-prick device, sharps box, test strip (ensure it is in date and matches the calibration code for the glucometer), gauze swab or similar.

Figure 7.3 Blood glucose measurement device or glucometer.

Figure 7.4 Blood glucose measurement: using the finger-prick device, stab the side of the finger.

- Wash and dry your hands and don gloves.

- Discuss the procedure with the patient – he may be able to advise on his normal blood glucose measurement and also on the best site to obtain the blood sample from. It would be helpful to choose an alternative site to one which was last used (the skin can become sore).

- Ensure that the finger being used is clean and dry (dirt contamination could affect the result).

- Using the finger-prick device, stab the side of the finger (less painful than the centre) to draw blood (Figure 7.4) and dispose of the sharp safely in the sharps box.

- Allow a droplet of blood to form (gentle squeezing may be necessary) onto the test strip following the manufacturer's recommendations.

- Apply gauze to puncture site and press to stop the bleeding; some patients will like to a plaster, some will not.

- Wait for the reading to be displayed on the glucometer (Figure 7.5), documenting the result.

MANAGEMENT OF ADRENAL INSUFFICIENCY

Adrenal insufficiency is a potentially fatal condition resulting from inadequate secretion of cortisol and/or aldosterone (Boon *et al.*, 2007). It can be associated with prolonged corticosteroid therapy and can persist for years after stopping.

ENDOCRINE DISORDERS

Figure 7.5 Blood glucose measurement: wait for the reading to be displayed on the glucometer.

A patient with adrenal insufficiency, when attending for dental treatment, may become very stressed, which could lead to hypotension and shock (British Medical Association & Royal Pharmaceutical Society, 2008).

Causes

Adrenal insufficiency can result from:

- *Primary adrenal insufficiency:* results from adrenal damage, e.g. Addison's disease;
- *Secondary adrenal insufficiency:* results from adrenocorticotrophic hormone (ACTH) deficiency due to pituitary or hypothalamic damage;
- Abrupt withdrawal of therapeutic steroid therapy can also cause ACTH deficiency.
- Stress, e.g. attending for dental treatment.

Clinical features

Clinical features include:

- shock, e.g. hypotension, tachycardia and pallor;
- anorexia;
- nausea and vomiting;

- abdominal pain;

- pyrexia;

- fatigue and lethargy.
  (Kearney & Dang, 2007).

Treatment

- Assess the patient following the ABCDE approach described in chapter 3.

- Call 999 for an ambulance.

- Lie the patient flat in the dental chair.

- Administer high flow oxygen using a non-rebreathe mask (see pages 37–9). If available, establish oxygen saturation monitoring using a pulse oximeter.

CONCLUSION

Endocrine disorders can be encountered in the dental practice. The management of hypoglycaemia in the dental practice has been discussed including blood glucose measurement. The management of the adrenal insufficiency has also been outlined.

REFERENCES

Bolli G, De Feo P, Compagnucci P *et al.* (1983) Abnormal glucose counter-regulation in insulin-dependent diabetes mellitus: interaction of anti-insulin antibodies and impaired glucagon and epinephrine secretion. *Diabetes*; 32:134–141.

Boon N, Colledge N, Walker B, Hunter J (2006) *Davidson's Principles & Practice of Medicine*, 20th edn. Churchill Livingstone, Edinburgh.

British Medical Association & Royal Pharmaceutical Society of Great Britain (2008) *BNF 56*. BMJ Publishing, London.

Diabetes UK (2009) www.diabetes.org.uk (accessed 24 July 2009).

Kearney T, Dang C (2007) Diabetic and endocrine emergencies. *Postgraduate Medical Journal*; 83(976):79–86.

Kubiak T, Kuhr B, Inselmann D, Hermanns N, Haak T (2004) Reversible cognitive deterioration after a single episode of severe hypoglycaemia. *Diabetic Medicine*; 21:1366–1367.

McLaren E, Somerville J (1988) Early warning symptoms of hypoglycaemia in ambulant diabetics. *Practical Diabetes*; 5:207–208.

Müller M, Hänsel M, Stehr S *et al.* (2008) A state-wide survey of medical emergency management in dental practices: incidence of emergencies and training experience. *Emergency Medicine Journal*; 25:296–300.

Resuscitation Council (UK) (2006) *Medical emergencies and resuscitation standards for clinical practice and training for dental practitioners and dental care professionals in general dental practice*. Resuscitation Council (UK), London.

Sampson M, Mortley S, Aldridge V (2006) The East Anglian Ambulance Trust diabetes emergencies audit: numbers and demographics. *Diabetes Medicine*; 23:101.

Shirayama H, Ohshiro Y, Kinjo Y *et al.* (2004) Acute brain injury in hypoglycaemia-induced hemiplegia. *Diabetic Medicine*; 21:623–624.

Shorr R, Ray W, Daugherty J *et al.* (1997) Incidence and risk factors for serious hypoglycaemia in older persons using insulin or sulfonylureas. *Archives of Internal Medicine*; 157:1681–1686.

Wyatt J, Illingworth R, Graham C *et al.* (2006) *Oxford Handbook of Emergency Medicine*, 3rd edn. Oxford University Press, Oxford.

ENDOCRINE DISORDERS

Chapter 8
Anaphylaxis

Anaphylaxis is an acute, severe, hypersensitivity reaction that can lead to asphyxia, cardiovascular collapse and cardiac arrest. In the general population, the incidence of anaphylaxis is on the increase (Department of Health, 2006), probably associated with a notable increase in the prevalence of allergic diseases in the last 30 years (Working Group of the Resuscitation Council (UK), 2008).

Anaphylaxis in the dental practice is very rare, accounting for approximately 1% of all encountered emergencies (Müller *et al.*, 2008). It may follow the administration of a drug, e.g. local anaesthetic, or exposure to a substance such as latex (Resuscitation Council (UK), 2006).

Anaphylaxis is often poorly managed; in particular, adrenaline is greatly under-used. The Resuscitation Council (UK) has published guidelines on the emergency management of anaphylaxis (Working Group of the Resuscitation Council (UK), 2008).

The aim of this chapter is to understand the emergency management of anaphylaxis.

LEARNING OUTCOMES

At the end of the chapter the reader will be able to:

- Define anaphylaxis
- Discuss the incidence of anaphylaxis
- Discuss the pathophysiology of anaphylaxis
- List the causes of anaphylaxis
- Describe the clinical features and diagnosis of anaphylaxis
- Discuss the treatment of anaphylaxis

DEFINITION

Anaphylaxis can be defined as 'a severe, life-threatening, generalised or systemic hypersensitivity reaction' (Johansson *et al.*, 2004). Basically, it is a life-threatening allergic reaction – the extreme end of the allergic spectrum (Anaphylaxis Campaign, 2009).

INCIDENCE

The incidence of anaphylaxis is on the increase (Gupta *et al.*, 2007), probably associated with a notable increase in the prevalence of allergic diseases in the last 30 years (Working Group of the Resuscitation Council (UK), 2008). A review of the literature (Jevon, 2008) on the incidence of anaphylaxis shows that:

- The incidence of anaphylaxis in the general population has increased;

- Since 1990, admissions for anaphylaxis have increased by 700% (Gupta *et al.*, 2007);

- In England, between 1990–91 and 2000–01, 13,230 people were admitted to hospital with anaphylaxis (Gupta *et al.*, 2003);

- Between 1991 and 1994 the number of discharges from hospitals in England with a diagnosis of anaphylaxis doubled from 415 to 876 (Sheikh & Alves, 2000);

- In 2004, 3171 patients were admitted to hospital with anaphylaxis (Peng & Jick, 2004);

- Anaphylaxis is more common in females than in males: in 2004, 58% of attendees to emergency departments with anaphylaxis were female, 42% were male (Peng & Jick, 2004); Webb and Lieberman (2006)'s findings were comparable: 62% females and 38% males;

- Mean age of patient with anaphylaxis is 37 years (Webb & Lieberman, 2006);

- Approximately 1 in 3,500 emergency department attendances are due to anaphylaxis (Stewart & Ewan, 1996);

- 50% of all anaphylactic reactions in the community are treated in hospital, with 20% requiring admission (Uguz *et al.*, 2005);

- Death from anaphylaxis is becoming more common, particularly in children and young adults (Ewan, 2000);

- In a survey of 620 dental surgeries, 7 had encountered anaphylaxis in the previous 12-month period (Müller *et al.*, 2008).

ANAPHYLAXIS

PATHOPHYSIOLOGY

Irrespective of the mechanism of anaphylaxis, mast cells and basophils release histamines and other vasoactive mediators which produce circulatory, respiratory, gastrointestinal and cutaneous effects (Wyatt *et al.*, 2006). These effects can include the development of pharyngeal and laryngeal oedema, bronchospasm, decreased vascular tone and capillary leak causing circulatory collapse (Jevon, 2004).

CAUSES

Causes of anaphylaxis include:

- drugs, e.g. penicillin, aspirin, local anaesthetic, surface anaesthetics (e.g. benzocaine);
- bee/wasp stings;
- foods, e.g. peanuts, tomatoes, fish;
- latex.
  (British Medical Association & Royal Pharmaceutical Society, 2008; Jevon, 2008; Anaphylaxis Campaign, 2009).

Anaphylaxis can also be associated with additives and excipients (an excipient is an inactive substance that serves as a vehicle or medium for a drug (Soanes & Stevenson, 2006)). It is therefore recommended to check the full formula of preparations, including those for topical application, especially those intended for use in the mouth (British Medical Association & Royal Pharmaceutical Society, 2008).

In approximately 40% of anaphylactic reactions, the cause is unknown (idiopathic anaphylaxis) (Webb & Lieberman, 2006; Greenberger, 2007).

CLINICAL FEATURES AND DIAGNOSIS

The lack of a consistent clinical picture can sometimes make an accurate diagnosis difficult (Project Team of the Resuscitation Council (UK), 2005). Anaphylaxis can vary in severity and the process can be slow, rapid or biphasic; occasionally the onset may be delayed by a few hours and even persist for longer than 24 hours (Fisher, 1986). As soon as possible a detailed history should be taken and the patient examined. The clinical presentation often includes:

- urticaria – a rash of round, red weals on the skin which itch intensely; sometimes referred to as nettlerash or hives (Soanes & Stevenson, 2006) (Figure 8.1);

ANAPHYLAXIS

Figure 8.1 Urticaria. Reproduced from Buxton PK, Morris-Jones R (2009) *ABC of Dermatology*, 5th edn. With permission from Wiley-Blackwell.

Figure 8.2 Angioedema. Reproduced from Buxton PK, Morris-Jones R (2009) *ABC of Dermatology*, 5th edn. With permission from Wiley-Blackwell.

- angioedema (facial swelling) (Figure 8.2);
- respiratory distress;
- wheeze/stridor;
- cardiovascular shock;
- tachycardia and hypotension;
- pallor.
  (Jevon, 2008; Anaphylaxis Campaign, 2009).

Anaphylaxis can vary in severity and the onset is usually rapid; occasionally it may be delayed by a few hours and may even persist for longer than 24 hours (Fisher, 1986). The patient feels unwell, usually has skin changes, e.g.

ANAPHYLAXIS

urticaria, and angioedema and will have a compromised airway and/or breathing and/or circulation (Jevon, 2008). Death from anaphylaxis usually occurs within 10–15 minutes, with cardiovascular collapse the commonest cause of death (Resuscitation Council (UK), 2006).

It is possible to mistake a panic attack or a vasovagal attack for anaphylaxis and adrenaline has been administered inappropriately in these situations (Johnston *et al.*, 2003). The clinical features of these presentations (Jevon, 2008) include:

- *Panic attack:* hyperventilation, tachycardia and anxiety-related erythematous (red) rash, but no hypotension, pallor, wheeze or urticarial rash;

- *Vasovagal attack:* relating to or denoting a temporary fall in blood pressure, with pallor, collapse, sweating and nausea, caused by overactivity of the vagus nerve particularly as a result of stress (Soanes & Stevenson, 2006): the absence of a rash, tachycardia and dyspnoea should rule out anaphylaxis as the cause of the collapse.

TREATMENT

The Resuscitation Council (UK) algorithm for the treatment of anaphylaxis in adults in the community is detailed in Figure 8.3. The treatment of anaphylaxis is as follows (Working Group of the Resuscitation Council (UK), 2008):

- Assess the patient following the ABCDE approach described in chapter 3.

- Call for help from colleagues.

- If able, stop or remove the probable cause of the anaphylaxis, e.g. remove latex gloves.

- Recline the patient into a position of comfort (the supine position may be helpful in hypotension but unhelpful in respiratory distress). If the patient is in shock it will be helpful to raise his legs.

- Ensure the patient has a clear airway; if stridor is present, alert senior expert help immediately (in anaphylaxis, stridor is probably due to potentially life-threatening laryngeal oedema).

- Administer high flow oxygen using a non-rebreathe mask (see pages 37–9). If available, establish oxygen saturation monitoring using a pulse oximeter.

- Closely monitor the patient's vital signs.

- Assess and re-assess the patient following the ABCDE approach.

ANAPHYLAXIS

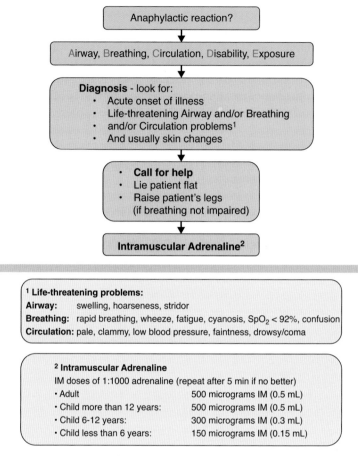

ANAPHYLAXIS

Figure 8.3 Resuscitation Council (UK) Algorithm for the management of anaphylaxis. Reproduced with kind permission from Resuscitation Council (UK).

- Repeat the adrenaline after 5 minutes if there is no improvement.

- Do not sit the patient up or stand him up if he is feeling faint or dizzy – he may be in profound shock and may then have a cardiac arrest.

Adrenaline

Adrenaline (Figure 8.4) is the most important drug in anaphylaxis (Fisher, 1995). To be effective, it needs to be administered promptly (Patel *et al.*, 1994). Adrenaline:

- reverses peripheral vasodilation;

- reduces oedema;

- dilates the airways;

- increases myocardial contractility;

- suppresses histamine and leukotriene release.

Figure 8.4 Adrenaline 1:1000 solution (1 mg in 1 ml).

The recommended dose of adrenaline is 500 μg (0.5 ml of 1:1000 solution) intramusculary (thigh) (British Medical Association & Royal Pharmaceutical Society, 2008). This can be repeated after 5 minutes if there is no clinical improvement (Resuscitation Council (UK), 2005); several doses may be required (British Medical Association & Royal Pharmaceutical Society, 2008). The intramuscular route for the administration of adrenaline should be used as it is relatively safe and adverse effects are rare. The only reported severe adverse effect following intramuscular administration of adrenaline was a myocardial infarction in a patient with severe ischaemic heart disease (Saff *et al.*, 1993).

Cautions include the following:

- Two strengths of adrenaline are available: 1:1000 solution is used for intramuscular injection, while the 1:10,000 solution, which some dental practices stock, is used for intravenous injection during cardiopulmonary resuscitation (Jevon, 2008).

- The subcutaneous route for the administration of adrenaline should not be utilised because absorption is considerably slower (Simons *et al.*, 1998).

Figure 8.5 EpiPen. Reproduced with kind permission from Alk-Abello UK.

ANAPHYLAXIS

EpiPen

If the patient has an EpiPen (Figure 8.5), this is considered an acceptable alternative if immediately available (Resuscitation Council (UK), 2006). This self-injector device comes in two preparations:

- 300 μg single dose: for adults and children over 30 kg (aged approximately 11+ years)
- 150 μg single dose: for children 15–30 kg (aged approximately 4–11 years) (British Medical Association & Royal Pharmaceutical Society, 2008).

Guidelines for using an EpiPen are given in Box 8.1.

Inhaled beta-2 agonist

Consider further bronchodilatory therapy, e.g. salbutamol inhaler (Working Group of the Resuscitation Council (UK), 2008).

Box 8.1   Procedure for using an EpiPen. Reproduced with kind permission from Alk-Abello UK.

INSTRUCTIONS FOR USE
EpiPen® adrenaline (Epinephrine) Auto-Injector:

Fig. 1

▶ Grasp EpiPen® in dominant hand, with thumb closest to grey safety cap

▶ With other hand, pull off **grey safety cap** (Fig. 1)

Fig. 2

▶ Jab firmly into outer thigh, through clothing if necessary (Fig. 2)

Fig. 3

10 Sec

▶ Hold in place for 10 seconds (Fig. 3)

▶ Massage injection area for 10 seconds

ALK
ABELLÓ

ANAPHYLAXIS

CONCLUSION

Anaphylaxis can be life threatening. This chapter has detailed the guidelines issued by the Resuscitation Council (UK) to treat it (Working Group of the Resuscitation Council (UK), 2008). Early treatment with intramuscular adrenaline is paramount.

REFERENCES

Allergy UK (2009) www.allergyuk.org (accessed 01/02/09).

Anaphylaxis Campaign (2009) www.anaphylaxis.org.uk (accessed 01/02/09).

British Medical Association & Royal Pharmaceutical Society of Great Britain (2008) *BNF 56*. BMJ Publishing, London.

Department of Health (2006) *A review of services for allergy: The epidemiology, demand for, and provision of treatment and effectiveness of clinical interventions.* Department of Health, London.

Ewan P (2000) Anaphylaxis. In Durham S (ed.) *ABC of Allergies*. BMJ Books, London.

Fisher M (1986) Clinical observations on the pathophysiology and treatment of anaphylactic cardiovascular collapse. *Anaesthesia and Intensive Care*; 14:17–21.

Fisher M (1995) Treatment of acute anaphylaxis. *BMJ*; 311:731–733.

Greenberger P (2007) Idiopathic anaphylaxis. *Immunology and Allergy Clinics of North America*; 27(2):273–293.

Gupta R, Sheikh A, Strachan D, Anderson H (2003) Increasing hospital admissions for systemic allergic disorders in England: an analysis of national admissions data. *BMJ*; 327:1142–1143.

Gupta R, Sheikh A, Strachan D, Anderson H (2007) Time trends in allergic disorders in the UK. *Thorax*; 62:91–96.

Jevon P (2004) *Anaphylaxis: A practical guide*. Butterworth Heinemann, Oxford.

Jevon P (2008) Severe allergic reaction: management of anaphylaxis in hospital. *British Journal of Nursing*; 17(2):104–108.

Johansson S, Bieber T, Dhal R et al. (2004) Revised nomenclature for allergy for global use: Report of the Nomenclature Review Committee of the World Allergy Organization, October 2003. *Journal of Allergy and Clinical Immunology*; 113(5):832–836.

Johnston S, Unsworth J, Gompels M (2003) Adrenaline given outside the context of life-threatening allergic reactions. *BMJ*; 326(7389):589–590.

Müller M, Hänsel M, Stehr S et al. (2008) A state-wide survey of medical emergency management in dental practices: incidence of emergencies and training experience. *Emergency Medicine Journal*; 25; 296–300.

Patel L, Radivan FS, David TJ (1994) Management of anaphylactic reactions to food. *Archives of Disease in Childhood*; 71:370–375.

Peng M, Jick H (2004) A population-based study of the incidence, cause and severity of anaphylaxis in the United Kingdom. *Archives of Internal Medicine*; 164(3):317–319.

Project Team of the Resuscitation Council (UK) (2005) *Emergency medical treatment of anaphylactic reactions*. Resuscitation Council (UK), London.

Resuscitation Council (UK) (2006) *Advanced Life Support*, 5th edn. Resuscitation Council (UK), London.

Saff R, Nahhas A, Fink J (1993) Myocardial infarction induced by coronary vasospasm after self-administration of epinephrine. *Annals of Allergy*; 70:396–398.

Sheikh A, Alves B (2000) hospital admissions for acute anaphylaxis: time trend study. *BMJ*; 320:1441.

Simons F, Roberts J, Gu X, Simons K (1998) Epinephrine absorption in cildrenwith a history of anaphylaxis. *Journal of Allergy and Clinical Immunology*; 101:33–37.

Soanes C, Stevenson A (2006) *Oxford Dictionary of English*, 2nd edn. Oxford University Press, Oxford.

Stewart A, Ewan P (1996) The incidence, aetiology and management of anaphylaxis presenting to an Accident & Emergency Department. *QJM*; 89:859–864.

Uguz A, Lack G, Pumphrey R *et al.* (2005) Allergic reactions in the community: a questionnaire survey of members of the anaphylaxis campaign. *Clinical and Experimental Allergy*; 35(6):746–750.

Webb L, Lieberman P (2006) Anaphylaxis: a review of 601 cases. *Annals of Allergy, Asthma, & Immunology*; 97(1):39–43.

Working Group of the Resuscitation Council (UK) (2008) *Emergency treatment of anaphylactic reactions: Guidelines for healthcare providers.* Resuscitation Council (UK), London.

Wyatt J, Illingworth R, Graham C *et al.* (2006) *Oxford Handbook of Emergency Medicine*, 3rd edn. Oxford University Press, Oxford.

ANAPHYLAXIS

Chapter 9

Cardiopulmonary resuscitation in the dental practice

INTRODUCTION

Cardiopulmonary arrest accounts for 0.3% of all medical emergencies encountered in the dental practice (Müller *et al.*, 2008). A recent study showed that cardiopulmonary arrest occurs in one in approximately 300,000 patients (Müller *et al.*, 2008).

Effective cardiopulmonary resuscitation (CPR) and early defibrillation are the only two interventions that have been shown to improve survival following a cardiopulmonary arrest: attention must therefore be focused on these while undertaking cardiopulmonary resuscitation (Nolan *et al.*, 2005). Following guidance from the Resuscitation Council (UK) (2006a), dental practices are purchasing automated external defibrillators (AEDs), thus enabling defibrillation before the arrival of the ambulance (if indicated). The procedure for using an AED is discussed in detail in chapter 11. The principles of airway management and ventilation are discussed in detail in chapter 10.

The aim of this chapter is to understand the procedure for cardiopulmonary resuscitation in the dental practice.

LEARNING OUTCOMES

At the end of the chapter the reader will be able to:

- Discuss the background to the Resuscitation Council (UK) automated external defibrillation algorithm
- Outline the procedure for cardiopulmonary resuscitation in the chair
- Discuss the principles of chest compressions

RESUSCITATION COUNCIL (UK) AUTOMATED EXTERNAL DEFIBRILLATION ALGORITHM

Ventricular fibrillation (see page 151) is the commonest primary arrhythmia at the onset of an adult cardiac arrest outside hospital (Jevon, 2009).

It is an eminently treatable rhythm with most eventual survivors coming from this group (Tunstall-Pedoe et al., 1992). Early defibrillation is the definitive treatment; the chances of success decline substantially with each passing minute. This process can be slowed, but not halted, by effective basic life support (Resuscitation Council (UK), 2006b). Effective CPR and defibrillation within 3–5 minutes of the onset of cardiac arrest can produce survival rates as high as 50–75% (Handley et al., 2005).

The Resuscitation Council (UK) automated external defibrillation algorithm (Figure 9.1) therefore focuses on the need to minimise any delay between the onset of cardiac arrest and defibrillation, if it is required. Until an AED is attached, only the first part of the algorithm will be followed (up to CPR 30:2). Hopefully, the dental practice will have immediate access to an AED, thus facilitating its early attachment and, if indicated, rapid defibrillation. Otherwise, CPR 30:2 will need to be performed while awaiting the emergency ambulance.

Modern AEDs will be programmed to follow the current Resuscitation Council (UK) automated external defibrillation algorithm (Resuscitation Council (UK), 2006a). Some older AEDs will follow previous (pre December 2005) guidelines. Some of these devices can be simply updated in line with the current guidelines (usually with an inexpensive item of software); others will not. If the latter is the case, the user should follow the AED's instructions (Resuscitation Council (UK), 2006c).

The automated external defibrillation algorithm is designed to be an aide-memoire, reminding the practitioner of the important aspects of assessment and treatment of cardiac arrest. It is not designed to be comprehensive or limiting. Each step that follows in the algorithm assumes that the previous one has been unsuccessful. Looping the algorithm reinforces the concept of constant assessment and reassessment.

PROCEDURE FOR CARDIOPULMONARY RESUSCITATION IN THE DENTAL CHAIR

The procedures described below and the sequences in which the actions are carried out are based on Resuscitation Council (UK) (2006a,b) recommendations and the automated external defibrillation algorithm. When more than one dental practitioner is present some of the actions described will be undertaken simultaneously. The main emphasis is on establishing as soon as possible

CARDIOPULMONARY RESUSCITATION
IN THE DENTAL PRACTICE

Figure 9.1 Resuscitation Council (UK) automated external defibrillation algorithm. Reproduced with kind permission from Resuscitation Council (UK).

whether defibrillation is required. Guidelines for safe handling during CPR should be followed (Resuscitation Council (UK), 2001) (see pages 10–11).

The following procedure also applies if the patient collapses on the floor, but with some modifications, e.g. chest compression technique (see pages 123–6) and ventilation technique (see pages 141–3).

Patient collapses in the dental chair

If the patient collapses in the dental chair, check whether he is responsive: gently shake his shoulders and ask him loudly 'are you alright?' (Figure 9.2).

Figure 9.2 CPR: assess responsiveness – shake and shout.

- *Patient responsive:* try and establish the cause of the collapse. The most likely cause is a vasovagal syncope (see pages 72–4). It will probably be necessary to put the dental chair into a horizontal position.

- *Patient unresponsive:* follow the automated external defibrillation algorithm (Figure 9.1):

Unresponsive

- Call for help from colleagues following local protocol. For example, this may simply involve shouting 'help' or shouting a certain code word such as 'code red', pressing an emergency buzzer or sending a message via the computer system. It would be helpful if a colleague could fetch the emergency equipment and oxygen.

- If not already done, recline the dental chair into the horizontal position. It is possible on most dental chairs to press an emergency button on the chair to active this position.

Open airway

As the patient is unresponsive and appears to be lifeless, it is important to establish whether he has had a cardiopulmonary arrest. Open the airway and look for signs of life:

- Open the airway by tilting the head and lifting the chin.

- Ensure the airway is clear: it may be necessary to apply suction.

CARDIOPULMONARY RESUSCITATION IN THE DENTAL PRACTICE

Figure 9.3 CPR: assess for signs of normal breathing – look, listen and feel.

- While maintaining the head tilt and chin lift, assess for signs of normal breathing; look for chest movement (breathing or coughing), listen for breath sounds at the patient's mouth and feel for air on your cheek (Soar & Spearpoint, 2005) (Figure 9.3). During the first few minutes following a cardiac arrest the patient may be barely breathing and may be taking infrequent noisy gasps: do not mistake this for normal breathing (Handley *et al.*, 2005). Also look for movement and other signs of life (Resuscitation Council (UK), 2006b). Take no longer than 10 seconds to check for signs of normal breathing (Jevon, 2009).

Patient breathing normally

If necessary request assistance from senior colleagues; assess the patient following the ABCDE approach; administer oxygen if necessary (see chapter 3). An unresponsive patient who is breathing normally should usually be placed in the lateral position.

Not breathing normally

- Call 999 for an ambulance. Ideally a colleague should be doing this. It would be helpful if a member of the team (if numbers allow) could wait outside the dental practice looking out for the ambulance (a patient may be willing to do this).

- Send or fetch for AED. Ideally, colleagues should bring the AED and resuscitation equipment, while chest compressions are immediately started. Request the AED and resuscitation equipment.

Figure 9.4 CPR: chest compressions.

CPR 30:2

- Ensuring that the chair is a suitable height for chest compressions, start CPR, 30 compressions to 2 ventilations. Perform chest compressions (Figure 9.4) at a rate of 100 per minute. Safe and effective chest compression technique is described below.

- While performing chest compressions, ask colleagues to prepare for ventilation, e.g. inserting an oropharyngeal airway (see pages 133–6), and connecting high flow oxygen to the ventilatory device, e.g. pocket mask or self-inflating bag-mask device (see pages 139 and 142). It is important to ensure that a ventilatory device is always immediately available as healthcare personnel should not be expected to perform mouth-to-mouth ventilation.

- After 30 compressions, release the pressure on the chest but leave the hands in situ, while colleagues deliver two ventilations. The re-start chest compressions. Most dental practices have a self-inflating bag for ventilations: attached oxygen 10 litres per minute as soon as possible and follow the two-person technique (Figure 9.5). If there are only two practitioners initially present, one could perform chest compressions and then squeeze the bag, while the other holds the mask on and maintains an open airway (alternatively a pocket mask could be used). The practitioner holding the mask on should ideally be sitting on the dentist's stool. The techniques for airway and ventilation are described in detail in the next chapter.

Figure 9.5 CPR: two-person technique for ventilating using a self-inflating bag.

Until AED is attached

- Once the AED arrives, position it near the patient (e.g. on his lap), switch it on and apply large adhesive electrodes as instructed by the AED; CPR should ideally continue while this is being done (Figure 9.6). The procedure for using an AED is described in detail on pages 153–6.

AED assesses rhythm

- Once the AED starts to assess the rhythm (ECG), ask colleagues to momentarily stop CPR as movement may interfere with this assessment.

Shock advised

- If a shock is advised, the AED will charge up automatically. Request that colleagues stand clear of the patient and the dental chair and move oxygen away. Perform a visual check before pressing the shock button (the safety features associated with AED use are discussed on page 153).

1 shock 150–360 J biphasic or 360 J monophasic

- Deliver shock (usually involves pressing a flashing shock button (Figure 9.7), though some AEDs are fully automatic and do no require the operator to do this). The AED will automatically select the shock energy required.

Figure 9.6 Using the AED: once the AED arrives, switch it on and apply large adhesive electrodes.

Figure 9.7 Using the AED: deliver shock (usually involves pressing a flashing shock button).

CARDIOPULMONARY RESUSCITATION
IN THE DENTAL PRACTICE

Figure 9.8 Using the AED: after delivery of the shock, re-start chest compressions immediately as instructed by the AED. Ideally change over the person performing chest compressions.

Immediately resume CPR 30:2 for 2 min

- Immediately resume chest compressions 30:2 for two minutes (Figure 9.8). Only stop CPR if the patient starts to breathe normally or if the AED instructs you to because it is re-assessing the ECG.

No shock advised

- Immediately resume chest compressions 30:2 for two minutes. Only stop CPR if the patient starts to breathe normally or if the AED instructs you to because it is re-assessing the ECG.

Continue until the victim starts to breathe normally

- While looping the algorithm following the AED's instructions, if the patient starts to breath normally, stop CPR and reassess following the ABCDE approach described in chapter 3.

- Administer high concentration oxygen using a non-rebreathe mask (see pages 37–9).

- Ideally place the patient in the lateral position; it is normal practice to leave the AED attached in case the patient has a further cardiopulmonary arrest.

- Reassure the patient and ensure that next of kin have been informed (if not already done).

PROCEDURE FOR PERFORMING CHEST COMPRESSIONS

The Resuscitation Council (UK) (2006b) stresses the importance of chest compressions. On confirmation of cardiac arrest, chest compressions should be started immediately while colleagues call the emergency services and fetch the resuscitation equipment and AED.

Safer handling techniques

Before starting chest compressions, to minimise the risk of injury it is important to follow Resuscitation Council (UK) (2001) safer handling guidelines:

- Remove any environmental hazards.

- *Performing chest compressions on a patient in the dental chair*: chest compressions can be performed effectively in the dental chair (Yokoyama *et al.*, 2008), as long as the correct procedures are followed: ensure the chair is at a height which places the patient between the knee and mid-thigh of the person performing chest compressions; stand at the side of the chair with the feet shoulder-width apart, position the shoulders directly over the patient's sternum and keep the arms straight (Figure 9.9).

- *Performing chest compressions on a patient on the floor*: kneel in the high-kneeling position, at the side of the patient, level with his chest with the knees a shoulder-width apart; position the shoulders directly over the patient's sternum and keep the arms straight (Figure 9.10).

Figure 9.9 Chest compressions in the dental chair.

Figure 9.10 Chest compression on the floor.

Technique

Once the correct position has been adopted (see above):

- Place the one hand on the centre of the patient's chest (this equates to the middle of the lower half of the sternum) and then place the other on top (this is quicker than spending time on the 'rib margin' location method); do not apply pressure over the end of the sternum or the upper abdomen (Handley *et al.*, 2005).

- Interlock and extend the fingers to avoid applying pressure over the patient's ribs (Figure 9.11).

- Apply pressure to the sternum only; do not apply pressure to the ribs, the end of the sternum or the upper abdomen (Handley *et al.*, 2005).

- Position the shoulders directly vertical above the patient's sternum, straighten the arms and lock the elbows (Figure 9.12); ensure the back is not twisted.

- Compress the sternum 4–5 cm and, following each compression, allow the chest to completely recoil back to its normal position (Yannopoulos *et al.*, 2005), thus facilitating venous return.

Figure 9.11 Chest compressions: interlock the fingers.

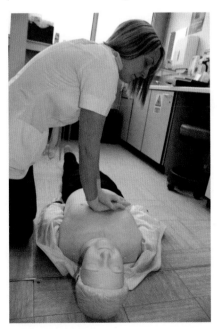

Figure 9.12 Chest compressions: position the shoulders directly vertical above the patient's sternum, straighten the arms and lock the elbows.

- Ensure that the force of compression results from flexing the hips (Resuscitation Council (UK), 2001).

- Perform chest compressions in a controlled manner; they should not be erratic or jerky.

- Continue chest compressions at a rate of 100/min (Jevon, 2009); this rate refers to the speed of compressions rather than the actual number delivered per minute; interruptions in chest compressions, e.g. to allow defibrillation, will result in fewer than 100 compressions being delivered in a minute.

- Ensure that the chest compression/chest relaxation phases are of equal duration.

- Ensure a ratio of 30 compressions: 2 ventilations (30:2) to allow more time for chest compressions. However, if the airway is secured with a tracheal tube (by the paramedic) asynchronous compressions and ventilations should be performed as this will result in a higher mean coronary perfusion pressure (a pause in chest compressions leads to a substantial fall in this pressure) (Resuscitation Council (UK), 2006b).

- To prevent fatigue, rotate the person performing chest compressions approximately every 2 minutes (Nolan *et al.*, 2005).

It is important to follow Resuscitation Council (UK) (2001) safer handling guidelines during CPR (see below). Ventilate using available airway and ventilation devices. Once the defibrillator arrives apply ECG leads/defibrillation.

CONCLUSION

Cardiopulmonary arrest in the dental practice is rare. If it does occur, it is important to follow Resuscitation Council (UK) guidelines (2006). In this chapter the Resuscitation Council (UK) automated external defibrillation algorithm has been outlined. The procedure for CPR in the chair and the principles of chest compressions have been discussed.

REFERENCES

Handley A, Koster R, Monsieurs K *et al.* (2005) Adult basic life support and use of automated external defibrillators. *Resuscitation*; 67: Suppl. S7–S23.

Jevon P (2009) *Advanced Cardiac Life Support*, 2nd edn. Wiley-Blackwell, Oxford.

Müller M, Hänsel M, Stehr S *et al.* (2008) A state-wide survey of medical emergency management in dental practices: incidence of emergencies and training experience. *Emergency Medicine Journal*; 25; 296–300.

Nolan J, Deakin C, Soar J *et al.* (2005) European Resuscitation Council Guidelines for Resuscitation 2005: Section 4. Adult advanced life support. *Resuscitation*; 675S,S39–S86.

Resuscitation Council (UK) (2001) *Guidance for Safer Handling during Resuscitation in Hospitals*. Resuscitation Council (UK), London.

Resuscitation Council (UK) (2006a) *Medical emergencies and resuscitation standards for clinical practice and training for dental practitioners and dental care professionals in general dental practice*. Resuscitation Council (UK), London.

Resuscitation Council (UK) (2006b) *Advanced Life Support*, 5th edn. Resuscitation Council (UK), London.

Resuscitation Council (UK) (2006c) *Statement on the use of Automated External Defibrillators (AEDs) until re-programming to be compliant with Guidelines 2005.* Resuscitation Council (UK), 2006.

Soar J, Spearpoint K (2005) In-hospital resuscitation. In Resuscitation Council (UK) *Guidelines 2005.* http://www.resus.org.uk/pages/inhresus.pdf (accessed 14/02/2009).

Tunstall-Pedoe H, Bailey L, Chamberlain D *et al.* (1992) Survey of 3765 cardiopulmonary resuscitations in British hospitals (the BRESUS study): methods and overall results. *BMJ* 304:1347–1351.

Yannopoulos D, Nadkarni V, McKnite S *et al.* (2005) Intrathoracic pressure regulator during continuous-chest-compression advanced cardiac resuscitation improves vital organ perfusion pressures in a porcine model of cardiac arrest. *Circulation*; 112:803–811.

Yokoyama T, Yoshida K, Suwa K (2008) Efficacy of external cardiac compression in a dental chair. *Resuscitation*; 79(1):175–176.

Chapter 10

Airway management and ventilation

INTRODUCTION

Failure of the circulation for three to four minutes (less if the patient is initially hypoxaemic) can lead to irreversible cerebral damage. Restarting the heart following a cardiac arrest may not be possible without adequate reoxygenation (Resuscitation Council (UK), 2006).

Patients who require resuscitation often have airway obstruction, usually secondary to loss of consciousness, but sometimes airway obstruction may be the primary cause of cardiorespiratory arrest (Nolan *et al.*, 2005). Airway obstruction can be subtle and is often undetected by healthcare professionals (Nolan *et al.*, 2005).

Dental practitioners must be competent at basic airway management and ventilation. Whatever the cause, prompt recognition and effective treatment of airway obstruction is essential, particularly during resuscitation as an open and clear airway is essential to help ensure adequate ventilation.

The aim of this chapter is to understand the principles of airway management and ventilation.

LEARNING OUTCOMES

At the end of the chapter the reader will be able to:

- List the causes of airway obstruction
- Outline the recognition of airway obstruction
- Describe simple techniques to open and clear the airway
- Discuss the use of an oropharyngeal airway
- Discuss the principles of ventilation
- Outline the treatment of foreign body airway obstruction

CAUSES OF AIRWAY OBSTRUCTION

Causes of airway obstruction include:

- *Displaced tongue* – causes include unconsciousness, sedation, cardiac arrest and trauma;
- *Fluid* – e.g. vomit, secretions and blood;
- *Foreign body* – e.g. dentures;
- *Laryngeal oedema* – causes include anaphylaxis and infection;
- *Bronchospasm* – causes include asthma, foreign body and anaphylaxis;
- *Pulmonary oedema* – causes include cardiac failure, anaphylaxis and near drowning (Jevon, 2006a).

RECOGNITION OF AIRWAY OBSTRUCTION

Whatever the cause of airway obstruction, prompt recognition and effective management are essential. Recognition is best achieved by following the familiar 'look, listen and feel' approach (Resuscitation Council (UK), 2006):

- *Look* for movements of the chest and abdomen;
- *Listen* at the mouth and nose for airflow;
- *Feel* at the mouth and nose for airflow.

Airway obstruction can be partial or complete, and can occur at any level from the nose and mouth down to the trachea (Jevon, 2006a).

Partial airway obstruction

Partial airway obstruction is usually characterised by noisy breathing:

- *Gurgling* – presence of fluid e.g. secretions in the main airways;
- *Snoring* – partial occlusion of the pharynx by the tongue;
- *Inspiratory stridor* – upper airway obstruction (at or above the level of the larynx), e.g. foreign body, laryngeal oedema;
- *Expiratory wheeze* – lower airway obstruction, e.g. asthma.

AIRWAY MANAGEMENT AND VENTILATION

Complete airway obstruction

Complete airway obstruction in a patient who is making respiratory efforts is characterised by paradoxical chest and abdominal movements ('see-saw' breathing) – on trying to breathe in, the chest is drawn inwards and the abdomen expands, the opposite happening when trying to breathe out (Resuscitation Council (UK), 2006). Use of accessory muscles, e.g. neck and shoulder muscles, may also be evident.

SIMPLE TECHNIQUES TO OPEN AND CLEAR THE AIRWAY

Head tilt, chin lift and jaw thrust are three manoeuvres that can improve the patency of the airway, which has been obstructed by the tongue or other upper airway structures, e.g. soft palate and epiglottis (Nolan *et al.*, 2005). As regurgitation of gastric contents and vomiting commonly occurs during resuscitation, suction is regularly required and proficiency in applying it is essential (Jevon, 2006a).

Head tilt, chin lift

The head tilt, chin lift manoeuvre (Figure 10.1) is considered the most effective method of opening the airway of an unconscious patient (Jevon, 2009). In basic life support it can achieve airway patency in 91% of cases (Guildner, 1976). By stretching the anterior tissues of the neck, it displaces the tongue forward away from the posterior pharyngeal wall and lifts the epiglottis from the laryngeal opening (Jevon, 2009). A cushion under the head and shoulders can help to maintain this position.

To perform head tilt and chin lift:

- Place the one hand on the patient's forehead and gently tilt the head back;
- Place the fingertips of the other hand under the point of the patient's chin and lift the chin upwards.
  (Jevon, 2006a).

Jaw thrust

The jaw thrust manoeuvre (Figure 10.2) is an alternative method to open the airway. It is recommended in patients with a suspected cervical spine injury (Jevon, 2009), as head tilt may aggravate the injury and damage the spinal cord (Donaldson *et al.*, 1997). When used in these patients, it should be accompanied

AIRWAY MANAGEMENT AND VENTILATION

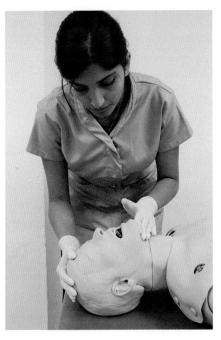

Figure 10.1 Head tilt, chin lift manoeuvre.

Figure 10.2 Jaw thrust manoeuvre.

by manual in-line immobilisation of the head and neck by an assistant (Lennarson *et al.*, 2001). However, if life-threatening airway obstruction persists, despite the application of effective jaw thrust or chin lift, head tilt should be performed gradually more and more until airway patency is achieved: the establishment of a clear airway takes priority over concerns about potential injury to the cervical spine (Nolan *et al.*, 2005).

AIRWAY MANAGEMENT AND VENTILATION

To perform a jaw thrust:

- Using the index fingers positioned just proximal to the angles of the jaw, displace the mandible anteriorly (together with the tongue);
- Using the thumbs, apply pressure on the chin to help open the mouth (Jevon, 2006a).

Suction

When obstruction is caused by vomit, secretions, etc., simple basic life support manoeuvres such as placing the patient in the lateral position and finger sweeps may help to clear the airway. The suction apparatus by the dental chair (Figure 10.3) can provide rapid suction of large volumes of fluid from the mouth and pharynx. A hand-held portable suction device (page 16) is useful for some situations, e.g. if the patient has collapsed in the waiting room.

Dentures

Well-fitting dentures should be left in place because they will help to maintain the normal shape of the face, facilitating an adequate seal when ventilating

Figure 10.3 Suction apparatus.

using a bag, valve or mask device. However, displaced or broken dentures should be removed (Nolan *et al.*, 2005).

USE OF OROPHARYNGEAL AIRWAY

The oropharyngeal airway is a useful adjunct because it can provide an artificial passage to airflow by separating the posterior pharyngeal wall from the tongue.

Oropharangeal airway

The oropharyngeal airway (Figure 10.4) can be used when there is obstruction of the upper airway due to the displacement of the tongue backwards and when glosso-pharyngeal and laryngeal reflexes are absent, e.g. during cardiopulmonary resuscitation.

Cautions

- An oropharyngeal airway should not be used in a patient who is not unconscious as it may induce vomiting and laryngospasm.
- An oropharyngeal airway should not be regarded as a definitive airway.
- The appropriate size of airway should always be estimated.
- The correct insertion technique should be adopted to minimise complications.

Figure 10.4 Oropharyngeal airway.

AIRWAY MANAGEMENT AND VENTILATION

Estimating the correct size

It is important to estimate the correct size. An oropharyngeal airway that is too big may occlude the airway by displacing the epiglottis (Jevon, 2009), may hinder the use of a face mask and may damage laryngeal structures, while one that is too small may occlude the airway by pushing the tongue back.

An appropriate sized airway is one that holds the tongue in the normal anatomical position and follows its natural curvature (Jevon, 2006b). The curved body of the oropharyngeal airway is designed to fit over the back of the tongue.

The correct size is one that equates to the vertical distance from the angle of the jaw to the incisors (Nolan *et al.*, 2005); this can be estimated by placing the airway against the face and measuring it from the patient's incisors to the angle of the jaw. A variety of different sizes are available, though normally sizes 2, 3 and 4 are adequate for small, medium and large adults, respectively (Resuscitation Council (UK), 2006).

Procedure for insertion

The correct insertion technique should be used in order to avoid unnecessary trauma to the delicate tissues in the mouth and so as not to inadvertently block the airway.

- Ensure the patient is in a supine position.

- Don gloves (if available).

- Clear the patient's airway, suction the mouth if necessary.

- Estimate the correct size by placing the airway against the patient's face and measuring it from the angle of the jaw to the incisors (Figure 10.5).

Figure 10.5 Insertion of oropharyngeal airway: estimating the correct size.

Figure 10.6 Insertion of oropharyngeal airway: insert the airway in the inverted position initially.

Figure 10.7 Insertion of oropharyngeal airway: as it passes over the soft palate, rotate the airway through 180 degrees.

- If possible, lubricate the airway before insertion (practically, in the emergency situation, this is rarely done).

- Open the patient's mouth, clear the airway by suction if necessary and insert the airway in the inverted position (Figure 10.6) (the curved part of the airway will help depress the tongue and prevent it from being pushed posteriorly).

- As it passes over the soft palate, rotate the airway through 180 degrees (Figure 10.7).

- After insertion, confirm that the airway has been position correctly: the patient's airway should be improved and the flattened reinforced section should be positioned between the patient's teeth, or between the gums if edentulous (Resuscitation Council (UK), 2006).

- Closely monitor the patency and position of the airway; it can become blocked by the tongue or epiglottis and can become wedged into the vallecula (Marsh *et al.*, 1991). Vomit, secretions and blood can also compromise its patency.

(source: Jevon, 2006b)

PRINCIPLES OF VENTILATION

> The most common cause of failure to ventilate is improper positioning of the head and chin (Jevon, 2006c)

Although chest compressions are now given priority over ventilations during the initial resuscitation sequence (Handley *et al.*, 2005), effective ventilations are still required and are indeed essential in prolonged arrests if cerebral function is to be maintained and the chance of survival is to be optimised.

There are three methods for ventilation:

- Mouth to mouth ventilation;

- Mouth to mask ventilation;

- Ventilation using a self-inflating bag (bag/valve/mask device).

Mouth to mouth ventilation

It should not be necessary to perform mouth-to-mouth resuscitation in the dental practice. At the very least a pocket mask should always be immediately available. However, for completeness, the procedure will now be described.

Mouth to mouth ventilation is a quick, effective way to provide adequate oxygenation and ventilation in a patient who is not breathing. However, it is only possible to deliver 16–17% oxygen to the patient; a ventilatory device with supplementary oxygen should be used as soon as practically possible.

Barrier devices

Both healthcare workers and laypersons are often reluctant to perform mouth to mouth ventilation, most commonly due to a fear of contracting HIV

(a)   (b)

Figure 10.8 (a) and (b) Barrier devices.

(Brenner *et al.*, 1997; Resuscitation Council (UK), 2006). Consequently a variety of barrier devices is available (Figure 10.8); facemasks with one-way valves prevent the transmission of bacteria, while face shields are less effective.

Procedure for mouth to mouth ventilation

1. Ensure the patient is supine. In a cardiac arrest, 30 chest compressions should have been performed first before delivering 2 ventilations (ratio 30:2) (Handley *et al.*, 2005).

2. Kneel in a comfortable position with the knees a shoulder width apart, at the side of the patient at the level of his nose and mouth (a wider base will be required to undertake compressions if only one person is performing CPR) (Resuscitation Council (UK), 2001).

3. Rest back to sit on the heels in the low kneeling position (Resuscitation Council (UK), 2001).

4. Apply a barrier device if one is available and if trained to do so.

5. Bend forwards from the hips, leaning down towards the patient's nose and mouth (Resuscitation Council (UK), 2001).

6. While maintaining head tilt and chin lift, pinch the soft part of the patient's nose (use the index finger and thumb of the hand on the patient's forehead), open the patient's mouth and take a normal breath in (Figure 10.9).

7. Place your lips around the patient's mouth, ensuring a good seal, and blow into the patient's mouth over 1 second and watch for chest to rise.

8. While still maintaining head tilt and chin lift, remove your mouth and watch for chest to fall. Repeat the procedure and then ensure 30 chest compressions are performed.

AIRWAY MANAGEMENT AND VENTILATION

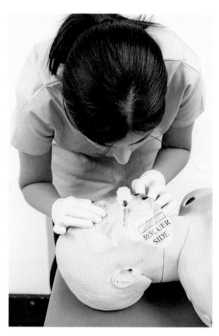

Figure 10.9 While maintaining head tilt and chin lift, pinch the soft part of the patient's nose (use the index finger and thumb of the hand on the patient's forehead), open the patient's mouth and take a normal breath in.

9. If the initial ventilation does not achieve chest rise as in normal breathing, before the next attempt, check the patient's mouth and remove any obstruction and recheck to ensure adequate head tilt and chin lift and ensure adequate seal. Only attempt 2 ventilations before 30 chest compressions are performed again (Handley *et al.*, 2005).

10. If the patient is in the dental chair (its height should already have been adjusted so that the patient is level between the knee and mid-thigh of the dental practitioner performing chest compressions): stand at the side facing the patient, level with his nose and mouth and bend forwards from the hips to minimise flexion of the spine; stand at the side facing the patient, level with his nose and mouth and bend forwards from the hips to minimise flexion of the spine (Resuscitation Council (UK), 2001).

(Resuscitation Council (UK), 2001, 2006; Jevon, 2006b)

Ineffective delivery of rescue breaths

If it difficult to deliver effective breaths:

- Ensure adequate head tilt and chin lift;
- Check the patient's mouth and remove any obstruction;

- Ensure a good seal between your mouth and the patient's mouth;

- Ensure the patient's nose is pinched during ventilation.

Minimising gastric inflation

Gastric inflation is commonly associated with mouth to mouth ventilation, occurring when the pressure in the oesophagus exceeds the opening pressure of the lower oesophageal sphincter, resulting in the sphincter opening (Jevon, 2009). During CPR, the oesophageal sphincter relaxes, thus increasing the likelihood of gastric inflation (Jevon, 2009).

Excessive tidal volumes or inspiratory flows can generate excessive airway pressures, which can lead to gastric inflation and the subsequent risk of regurgitation and aspiration of gastric contents (Nolan *et al.*, 2005). It is therefore recommended to deliver each ventilation over 1 second, with sufficient volume to achieve chest rise, but avoiding rapid and forceful ventilations (Handley *et al.*, 2005).

Mouth to mask ventilation (pocket mask)

The pocket mask (Figure 10.10) is an excellent first response device. It is transparent, thus enabling prompt detection of vomit or blood in the patient's airway. A one-way valve directs the patient's expired air away from the nurse.

Most pocket masks have an oxygen connector for the attachment of supplementary oxygen (10 litres/min) (Resuscitation Council (UK), 2006), enabling an inspired oxygen concentration of approximately 50% to be achieved. If there is no oxygen connector, supplementary oxygen can still be added by

Figure 10.10 Pocket mask.

AIRWAY MANAGEMENT AND VENTILATION

placing the oxygen tubing underneath one side of the mask and pressing down to achieve a seal (Nolan *et al.*, 2005).

Procedure for mouth to mask ventilation – patient on the floor

1. Don gloves (if available).

2. Kneel behind the patient's head, ensuring the knees are a shoulder-width apart (if working alone, kneel at the side of the patient level with his nose and mouth) (Resuscitation Council (UK), 2001).

3. Rest back to sit on the knees and adopt a low kneeling position (Resuscitation Council (UK), 2001).

4. Bend forwards from the hips, leaning down towards the patient's face and resting the elbows on your legs to support your weight (Resuscitation Council (UK), 2001).

5. If available, attach oxygen to the oxygen connector on the mask at a rate of 10 litres/minute (Resuscitation Council (UK), 2000). If there is no oxygen connector, place the oxygen tubing underneath one side of the mask and press down to achieve a seal (Nolan *et al.*, 2005).

6. Apply the mask to the patient's face; press down with the thumbs and lift the chin into the mask by applying pressure behind the angles of the jaw.

7. Take a breath in and ventilate the patient with sufficient air to cause visible chest rise (Figure 10.11). Each ventilation should last 1 second.

(Resuscitation Council (UK), 2001, 2006; Jevon, 2006b)

AIRWAY MANAGEMENT AND VENTILATION

Figure 10.11 Mouth to mask ventilation: take a breath in and ventilate the patient with sufficient air to cause visible chest rise.

Procedure for mouth to mask ventilation – patient in the dental chair

1. Don gloves (if available).

2. Ensure the patient is supine in the chair (its height should already have been adjusted so that the patient is level between the knee and mid-thigh of the person performing chest compressions).

3. While your colleague performs chest compressions, sit on the dentist's stool behind the head end of the chair, facing the patient.

4. If available, attach oxygen to the oxygen connector on the mask at a rate of 10 litres/minute (Resuscitation Council (UK), 2000). If there is no oxygen connector, place the oxygen tubing underneath one side of the mask and pressing down to achieve a seal (Nolan et al., 2005).

5. Apply the mask to the patient's face; press down with the thumbs and lift the chin into the mask by applying pressure behind the angles of the jaw.

6. Bend forwards from the hips, leaning down towards the patient's face and resting the elbows on your legs to support your weight (Resuscitation Council (UK), 2001).

7. Take a breath in and ventilate the patient with sufficient air to cause visible chest rise. Each ventilation should last 1 second.

8. Always adopt a comfortable position for ventilation and avoid static postures (Resuscitation Council (UK), 2001); ideally sit on the dentist's stool.

(Resuscitation Council (UK), 2001, 2006; Jevon, 2006b)

> If working alone when performing mouth to mask ventilation, stand at the side facing the patient, level with his nose and mouth, and bend forwards from the hips to minimise flexion of the spine (Resuscitation Council (UK), 2001)

AIRWAY MANAGEMENT AND VENTILATION

Bag-mask ventilation

The bag-mask (self-inflating bag) (Figure 10.12) device allows the delivery of higher concentrations of oxygen. If an oxygen reservoir bag is attached, with an oxygen flow rate of 10 litres per minute, an inspired oxygen concentration of approximately 85% can be achieved (Nolan et al., 2005).

However, its use by a single person requires considerable skill. When used with a face mask, it can be difficult to achieve a seal with the mask, maintain an open airway and squeeze the bag (Jevon, 2009). A two-person technique is

Figure 10.12 Self-inflating bag.

therefore recommended, one person to open the airway and ensure a good seal with the mask, while the other squeezes the bag (Nolan *et al.*, 2005).

Procedure for bag-mask ventilation – patient on the floor

1. Don gloves (if available).

2. Select an appropriately sized mask, i.e. one that comfortably covers the mouth and nose but does not cover the eyes or override the chin.

3. Ensure the oxygen reservoir bag is attached to the self-inflating bag and connect oxygen at a flow rate of 10 litres per minute (Nolan *et al.*, 2005).

4. Kneel behind the patient's head, ensuring the knees are a shoulder-width apart (Resuscitation Council (UK), 2001).

5. Rest back to sit on the heels and adopt a low kneeling position (Resuscitation Council (UK), 2001).

6. Rest your elbows on your legs to support your weight; adopt a comfortable position, e.g. bend forwards or remain upright (Resuscitation Council (UK), 2001).

7. Tilt the patient's head back, apply the mask to the face, pressing down on it with the thumbs. Lift the chin into the mask by applying pressure behind the angles of the jaw. An open airway and an adequate face to mask seal should now be achieved. A cushion under the head and shoulders can help to maintain this position.

8. Ask a colleague to kneel to the side, adopting the same stance as described above.

Figure 10.13 Patient on the floor: ventilation with a self-inflating bag.

9. After the delivery of 30 chest compressions, ask your colleague to deliver two ventilations, squeezing the self-inflating bag (not the oxygen reservoir bag) sufficiently to cause visible chest rise (Figure 10.13). Each ventilation should be delivered over 1 second.

10. Observe for chest rise and fall. If the chest does not rise, re-check the patency of the airway; slight readjustment may be all that is required.

11. Adopt a comfortable position for ventilation and avoid static postures. It may be helpful to support your weight by resting your elbows on the bed (Resuscitation Council (UK), 2001).

(Resuscitation Council (UK), 2001, 2006; Jevon, 2006b)

Procedure for bag-mask ventilation – patient in the dental chair

1. Don gloves (if available).

2. Ensure the patient is supine. The height of the chair should already have been adjusted so that the patient is level between the knee and mid-thigh of the person performing chest compressions (Resuscitation Council (UK), 2001).

AIRWAY MANAGEMENT AND VENTILATION

3. Adopt a comfortable position for ventilation. Sit on the dentist's stool behind the head end of the chair, facing the patient. It may be helpful to support your weight by resting your elbows on your knees (Resuscitation Council (UK), 2001).

4. Select an appropriately sized mask, i.e. one that comfortably covers the mouth and nose but does not cover the eyes or override the chin.

5. Ensure the oxygen reservoir bag is attached to the self-inflating bag and connect oxygen at a flow rate of 10 litres per minute (Nolan *et al.*, 2005).

6. Tilt the patient's head back, apply the mask to the face, pressing down on it with the thumbs. Lift the chin into the mask by applying pressure behind the angles of the jaw. An open airway and an adequate face to mask seal should now be achieved. A small cushion under the head and shoulders can help to maintain this position.

7. Ask a colleague to stand at the side facing the patient's head, with the feet in the walk/stand position (Resuscitation Council (UK), 2001).

8. After the delivery of 30 chest compressions, ask your colleague to deliver two ventilations, squeezing the self-inflating bag (not the oxygen reservoir bag) sufficiently to cause visible chest rise (Figure 10.14). Each ventilation should be delivered over 1 second.

9. Observe for chest rise and fall. If the chest does not rise, re-check the patency of the airway; slight readjustment may be all that is required.

10. Adopt a comfortable position for ventilation and avoid static postures. It may be helpful to support your weight by resting your elbows on the bed (Resuscitation Council (UK), 2001).

(Resuscitation Council (UK), 2001, 2006; Jevon, 2006b)

Figure 10.14 Patient in the dental chair: ventilation with a self-inflating bag.

Minimising gastric inflation

Excessive tidal volumes or inspiratory flows can generate excessive airway pressures, which can lead to gastric inflation and the subsequent risk of regurgitation and aspiration of gastric contents (Nolan *et al.*, 2005). It is therefore recommended to deliver each ventilation over 1 second, with sufficient volume to achieve chest rise, but avoiding rapid and forceful ventilations (Handley *et al.*, 2005).

Ineffective ventilations

If ventilations fail to achieve chest rise:

- ensure adequate head tilt and chin lift;
- recheck the patient's mouth and remove any obstruction;
- ensure there is a good seal between the mask and the patient's face.

TREATMENT OF FOREIGN BODY AIRWAY OBSTRUCTION

Foreign body airway obstruction (choking) is a life-threatening emergency. As most such events are associated with eating, they are commonly witnessed, thus providing an opportunity for early intervention while the patient is still conscious (Handley *et al.*, 2005). Case reports have demonstrated the effectiveness of back blows, abdominal thrusts and chest thrusts for the treatment of foreign body airway obstruction (ILCOR, 2005), successful treatment often requiring more than one particular intervention (Redding, 1979).

Incidence

Foreign body airway obstruction is an uncommon, yet potentially treatable, cause of accidental death (Fingerhut *et al.*, 1998). Each year in the UK approximately 16,000 adults and children receive treatment in the emergency department for foreign body airway obstruction (Handley *et al.*, 2005); less than 1% of these are fatal (Department of Trade & Industry, 1999a). In adults the commonest cause of foreign body airway obstruction is food, e.g. meat, poultry and fish (Department of Trade & Industry, 1999a); in children half of cases are caused by food (usually sweets) and half by such items as small toys and coins (Department of Trade & Industry, 1999b).

Recognition of foreign body airway obstruction

Complete foreign body airway obstruction is often characterised by a sudden inability to talk, maximal respiratory effort, development of cyanosis and clutching of the neck. In partial airway obstruction, the patient will be distressed, may cough and may have a wheeze. In complete airway obstruction, the casualty will be unable to speak, breathe or cough and will eventually collapse and become unconscious. Always ask the patient 'are you choking?' (Handley *et al.*, 2005). If he responds 'yes' by nodding his head without speaking, this indicates severe airway obstruction requiring urgent treatment (American Heart Association, 2005).

If the patient is choking, but able to breathe, encourage him to cough. If the patient is choking and is unable to breathe or is displaying signs of becoming weak or stops breathing or coughing, immediate intervention is required:

Procedure for treatment of foreign body airway obstruction

- Stand at side, slightly behind the patient.

- Support his chest with one hand and lean him well forward. This will help ensure that if the foreign body is dislodged, it will drop out of the mouth instead of slipping further down the airway.

- Deliver up to five back blows between the scapulae using the heel of the hand (Figure 10.15). After each back blow, check to see if it has been successful at relieving the obstruction.

Figure 10.15 Choking: back slaps.

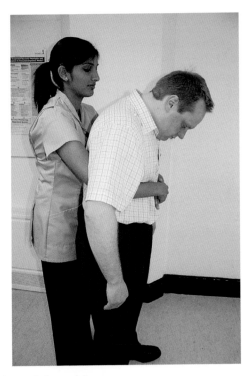

Figure 10.16 Choking: abdominal thrusts.

- If the back blows fail, proceed to abdominal thrusts.
- Stand behind the patient, placing both arms around his upper abdomen.
- Lean the patient forward.
- Place a clenched fist between the patient's umbilicus and xiphisternum and clasp it with the other hand (Figure 10.16).
- Deliver up to five sharp thrusts to the abdomen, inwards and upwards.
- If the obstruction remains, continue alternating five back blows with five chest abdominal thrusts.

If the patient loses consciousness:

- carefully support him to the ground;
- immediately call 999 for an ambulance;
- start CPR, 30 chest compressions first (even if there is a pulse) – chest compressions may relieve the obstruction (Handley *et al.*, 2005).

Chest thrusts v abdominal thrusts

Chest thrusts can generate higher airway pressures than abdominal thrusts (Guilder *et al.*, 1976; Ruben & Macnaughton, 1978). If a patient with a foreign body airway obstruction loses consciousness, CPR should be started, as chest thrusts are almost identical to chest compressions (Handley *et al.*, 2005). Then each time the airway is opened to provide ventilations, check the mouth in case the foreign body has been dislodged.

Finger sweeps

The routine use of a finger sweep to clear the airway in the absence of visible airway obstruction has yet to be evaluated (Hartrey & Bingham, 1995; Elam *et al.*, 1960). Finger sweeps have been reported to cause harm to both the patient (Resuscitation Council (UK), 2006) and the rescuer (ILCOR, 2005). Blind finger sweeps are not recommended; only manually remove a foreign body in the airway if it can be seen (Handley *et al.*, 2005).

Follow-up

Following successful treatment, a foreign body may still be present in the airways: therefore if the patient has dysphagia, has a persistent cough or complains of having something 'stuck in his throat', he should be referred to a doctor (Handley *et al.*, 2005).

As abdominal thrusts can cause serious internal injury, e.g. rupture or laceration of abdominal or thoracic viscera, patients who have been treated with abdominal thrusts must be referred to a doctor (ILCOR, 2005).

CONCLUSION

Effective airway management and ventilation are essential if oxygen supply to the brain is to be maintained during cardiopulmonary resuscitation. This chapter has described the principles of basic airway management and ventilation.

REFERENCES

American Heart Association (2005) 2005 American Heart Association Guidelines for Cardiopulmonary Resuscitation and Emergency cardiovascular care. *Circulation*; 112:24 suppl.

Brenner B, Van D, Cheng D, Lazar E (1997) Determinants of reluctance to perform CPR among residents and applicants: the impact of experience on helping behaviour. *Resuscitation*; 35:203–211.

Department of Trade & Industry (1999a) Choking. In *Home and leisure accident report*. Department of Trade & Industry, London.

Department of Trade & Industry (1999b) *Choking risks for children*. Department of Trade & Industry, London.

Donaldson W, Heil B, Donaldson V, Silvaggio V (1997) The effect of airway maneuvers on the unstable C1-C2 segment: a cadaver study. *Spine*; 22:1215–1218.

Elam J, Ruben A, Greene D (1960) Resuscitation of drowning victims. *JAMA*; 174:13–16.

Fingerhut L, Cox C, Warner M (1998) International comparative analysis of injury mortality: findings from the ICE on injury statistics. International collaborative effort on injury statistics. *Advance Data*; 12:1–20.

Guildner C, Williams D, Subitch T (1976) Airway obstructed by foreign material: the Heimlich maneuver. *JACEP*; 5:675–677.

Handley A, Koster R, Monsieurs K *et al.* (2005) European Resuscitation Council Guidelines for Resuscitation 2005: Section 2. Adult basic life support and use of automated external defibrillators. *Resuscitation*; 67S1, S7–S23.

Hartrey R, Bingham R (1995) Pharyngeal trauma as a result of blind finger sweeps in the choking child. *Journal of Accident and Emergency Medicine*; 12:52–54.

ILCOR (2005) Part 2 Adult basic life support 2005 international consensus on cardiopulmonary resuscitation and emergency cardiovascular care science with treatment recommendations. *Resuscitation*; 67:187–200.

Jevon P (2006a) Resuscitation skills – part 2: clearing the airway. *Nursing Times*; 102(26):26–27.

Jevon P (2006b) Resuscitation skills – part 3: basic airway management. *Nursing Times*; 102(27):26–27.

Jevon P (2006c) Mask ventilation. *Nursing Times*; 102(38):28–29.

Jevon P (2009) *Advanced Cardiac Life Support*, 2nd edn. Wiley-Blackwell, Oxford.

Lennarson P, Smith D, Sawin P *et al.* (2001) Cervical spine motion during intubation: efficacy of stabilization maneuvers in the setting of complete segmental instability. *Journal of Neurosurgery*; 94:265–270.

Marsh A, Nunn J, Taylor S, Charlesworth C (1991) Airway obstruction associated with the use of the Guedel airway. *British Journal of Anaesthesia*; 67:517–523.

Nolan J, Deakin C, Soar J *et al.* (2005) European Resuscitation Council Guidelines for Resuscitation 2005: Section 4. Adult advanced life support. *Resuscitation*; 675S, S39–S86.

Redding J (1979) The choking controversy: critique of evidence of the Heimlich maneuver. *Critical Care Medicine*; 7:475–479.

Resuscitation Council (UK) (2001) *Guidance for safer handling during resuscitation in hospitals*. Resuscitation Council (UK), London.

Resuscitation Council (UK) (2006) *Advanced Life Support Provider Manual*, 5th edn. Resuscitation Council (UK), London.

Ruben H, Macnaughton F (1978) The treatment of food-choking. *Practitioner*; 221:725–729.

AIRWAY MANAGEMENT AND VENTILATION

Chapter 11

Automated external defibrillation

INTRODUCTION

Defibrillation is the delivery of an electrical current across the myocardium of significant magnitude to depolarise a critical mass of the myocardium simultaneously to enable the restoration of organised electrical activity (Deakin & Nolan, 2005). A key component in the chain of survival (page 2), defibrillation is one of only two interventions that have been shown unequivocally to improve long-term survival following a cardiac arrest, the other being basic life support (Resuscitation Council (UK), 2006a).

The modern automated external defibrillator (AED) abolishes the need for the operator to have ECG interpretation skills. Spoken and/or visual prompts guide the operator through the safe use of the AED. As minimal training is required, it can be used by a wide range of personnel, including dental practice staff. The Resuscitation Council (UK) (2006b) now recommends that every dental practice should have immediate access to a defibrillator. If required, defibrillation should be undertaken by dental staff before the arrival of the paramedics.

The aim of this chapter is to understand the principles of automated external defibrillation.

LEARNING OUTCOMES

At the end of this chapter the reader will be able to:

- Recognise ventricular fibrillation
- Discuss the physiology of defibrillation
- Outline the factors affecting successful defibrillation
- Discuss the safety issues related to defibrillation
- Describe the procedure for automated external defibrillation

Figure 11.1 Ventricular fibrillation.

VENTRICULAR FIBRILLATION

'The cardiac pump is thrown out of gear, and the last of its vital energy is dissipated in a violent and prolonged turmoil of fruitless activity in the ventricular walls.' (McWilliam, 1889)

In ventricular fibrillation (Figure 11.1), the myocardium is depolarising at random resulting in uncoordinated electrical activity, with subsequent loss of cardiac output and cardiac arrest. Causes include myocardial ischaemia, electrolyte imbalance, hypothermia, drug toxicity and electric shock.

Ventricular fibrillation is the commonest primary arrhythmia at the onset of cardiac arrest in adults (Handley *et al.*, 2005). It is an eminently treatable arrhythmia with most eventual survivors of a cardiac arrest belonging to this group (Tunstall-Pedoe *et al.*, 1992).

Early defibrillation is the definitive treatment; the chances of success decline substantially (7–10%) with each passing minute of delay to defibrillation (Waalewijn *et al.*, 2001). There is a slower decline if there is adequate basic life support (Resuscitation Council (UK), 2006a).

PHYSIOLOGY OF DEFIBRILLATION

The heart can respond to an extrinsic electrical impulse just as it can respond to an impulse from the sinoatrial node or from an ectopic focus. It is thought that successful defibrillation occurs when a critical mass of myocardium is depolarised by the passage of an electric current (Resuscitation Council (UK), 2006a); if 75–90% of myocardial cells are in the repolarisation phase when the current is removed, successful defibrillation occurs and the sinoatrial node or another intrinsic pacemaker can then regain control.

Success will depend on the actual current flow rather than shock energy. This current flow is influenced by transthoracic impedance (resistance of the chest tissues), electrode position and shock energy delivered. Only a small proportion of the energy delivered actually reaches the myocardium; an effective defibrillation technique is essential to optimise the chances of successful defibrillation.

AUTOMATED EXTERNAL DEFIBRILLATION

FACTORS AFFECTING SUCCESSFUL DEFIBRILLATION

If defibrillation is to be successful, sufficient electrical current needs to pass through the chest and depolarise a critical mass of myocardium. Transthoracic impedance and incorrect positioning of the adhesive pad electrodes are two key factors that can affect successful defibrillation.

Transthoracic impedance

Transthoracic impedance is the resistance to the flow of current through the chest; the greater the resistance, the less the current flow. The contact between the adhesive pad electrodes and the skin can be poor if the patient has a hairy chest, trapping air between the electrode and the skin; this can result in increased transthoracic impedance, reduced defibrillation efficacy and arcing (sparks) causing burns to the patient's chest (Deakin & Nolan, 2005).

If the patient has a hairy chest and a razor is immediately available, quickly remove hair from the area where the adhesive pad electrodes are going to be placed, but if a razor is not immediately available, do not delay defibrillation (Resuscitation Council (UK), 2006a).

Incorrect positioning of the adhesive pad electrodes

The adhesive pad electrodes should be placed in the correct positions on the chest wall to maximise the current flow through the myocardium. It is important to follow the manufacturer's instructions – most adhesive pad electrodes will have a diagram to guide correct placement (Figure 11.2). Adhesive pad electrodes are generally placed, one on the anterior chest, just to the right of the sternum (not over the sternum) below the right clavicle, the other in the mid-axillary line near the apex of the heart. In women, breast tissue should be avoided as this can increase transthoracic impedance.

Figure 11.2 Adhesive pad electrodes.

AUTOMATED EXTERNAL DEFIBRILLATION

The accuracy of electrode placement by healthcare staff has been questioned, and care should be taken to ensure their correct placement following the manufacturer's instructions.

SAFETY ISSUES AND DEFIBRILLATION

General safety issues

- Confirm cardiac arrest.

- Avoid direct and indirect contact with the patient. All personnel should be well away from the dental chair; no one should be touching the patient or anything attached to the dental chair.

- Ensure that no personnel are standing in water which is in contact with the chair.

- Temporarily remove oxygen delivery device at least 1 metre away from the patient's chest (Resuscitation Council (UK), 2006a).

- Shout 'stand clear' and check all personnel are safely clear prior to defibrillation. No person should be touching the patient or anything in contact with the patient, e.g. bed or drip stand.

- Place the adhesive pad electrodes 12 to 15 cm away from an implanted pacing unit or implantable cardioverter defibrillator (ICD) (Resuscitation Council (UK), 2006a) (most units are sited below the left clavicle, therefore the standard electrode position can be adopted, if below the right clavicle the anterior-posterior paddle position may be necessary).

Safety issues when using adhesive electrode pads

- Ensure that electrode pads are in date.

- Ensure that the patient's chest is wiped dry.

- Shave the chest if necessary (see above).

PROCEDURE FOR AUTOMATED EXTERNAL DEFIBRILLATION

The following procedure for automated external defibrillation is based on Resuscitation Council (UK) (2006a) recommendations and the Resuscitation

AUTOMATED EXTERNAL DEFIBRILLATION

Council (UK) algorithm for automated external defibrillation (see Figure 9.1).

1. Confirm cardiac arrest and ensure a colleague calls 999 for ambulance; if numbers allow, ask someone to wait outside the dental practice to 'flag down' the ambulance.

2. Commence CPR: 30 chest compressions: 2 ventilations; request the resuscitation equipment and AED.

3. Switch on automated external defibrillator (AED) and follow spoken and/or visual prompts.

4. Expose the patients chest; remove GTN patches (Wrenn, 1990).

5. Prepare the patient's skin as necessary; ensure that the skin is dry and if necessary quickly remove any excess chest hair (if the patient has a hairy chest, the defibrillation electrodes may stick to the hairs resulting in high transthoracic impedance.

6. Apply adhesive pad electrodes to the patient's bare chest following the manufacturer's recommendations; the standard position for the position of the electrodes is one on the anterior chest, just to the right of the sternum (not over the sternum) below the right clavicle, the other in the mid-axillary line approximately level with the fifth intercostal space (Figure 11.3).

7. Stop CPR and ensure nobody is touching the patient during ECG analysis by the AED. This is to prevent artifactual errors during ECG analysis (Jevon, 2009). Some AEDs require the operator to press an 'analyse' button, while others automatically begin assessment once the adhesive pad electrodes are attached to the patient's chest.

Figure 11.3 Automated external defibrillation: application of adhesive pad electrodes on the chest.

Figure 11.4 Automated external defibrillation: if shock is advised, shout 'stand clear' and perform visual check to ensure that all staff are clear.

Figure 11.5 Automated external defibrillation: press shock button.

8. If shock is advised, shout 'stand clear' and perform visual check to ensure all staff are clear (Figure 11.4).

9. Check all personnel are safely clear before defibrillation. No person should be touching the patient or anything in contact with the patient, e.g. chair or equipment connected to the chair. Request that the ventilatory device and attached oxygen is temporarily removed 1 metre away from the patient (Resuscitation Council (UK), 2006a).

10. Press shock button as indicated (if the AED is fully automated, it will deliver the shock automatically) (Figure 11.5).

AUTOMATED EXTERNAL DEFIBRILLATION

11. Continue CPR 30 compressions : 2 ventilations as guided by the voice/visual prompts.

12. Following 2 minutes of CPR the AED will assess again (see step 7 on page 54). If a further shock is advised, repeat steps 8–11. If no shock is advised, repeat step 11 if there are no signs of life.

Implantable cardioverter defibrillator

If a patient with an implantable cardioverter defibrillator (ICD) has a cardiac arrest, standard CPR can be carried out without any risks to the team. If the ICD discharges it will not be detected by those carrying out the CPR. Place the adhesive pad electrodes 12 to 15 cm away from an implanted pacing unit or implantable cardioverter defibrillator (ICD) (Resuscitation Council (UK), 2006) (most units are sited below the left clavicle, therefore the standard electrode position can be adopted, if below the right clavicle the anterior-posterior paddle position may be necessary).

CONCLUSION

Early defibrillation is a key component in the chain of survival. It has been shown unequivocally to improve long-term survival following a cardiac arrest. It should be delivered promptly, safely and effectively. The Resuscitation Council (UK) (2006a) recommends that dental practices should have immediate access to an AED. The principles of automated external defibrillation have been described.

REFERENCES

Deakin C, Nolan J (2005) European Resuscitation Council guidelines for resuscitation 2005: Section 3. Electrical therapies: automated external defibrillators, defibrillation, cardioversion and pacing. *Resuscitation*; 675S:S25–S37.

McWilliam J (1899) Cardiac failure and sudden death. *BMJ*; I:6–8.

Resuscitation Council (UK) (2006a) *Advanced Life Support*, 5th edn. Resuscitation Council (UK), London.

Resuscitation Council UK (2006b) *Medical emergencies and resuscitation standards for clinical practice and training for dental practitioners and dental care professionals in general dental practice*. Resuscitation Council (UK), London.

Tunstall-Pedoe H, Bailey L, Chamberlain D *et al.* (1992) Survey of 3765 cardiopulmonary resuscitations in British hospitals (the BRESUS study): methods and overall results. *BMJ* 304:1347–1351.

Waalewijn R, de Vos R, Tijssen J, Koster R (2001) Survival models for out-of-hospital cardiopulmonary resuscitation from the perspectives of the bystander, the first responder and the paramedic. *Resuscitation*; 51:113–122.

Wrenn K (1990) The hazards of defibrillation through nitroglycerin patches. *Annals of Emergency Medicine*; 19:1327–1328.

Chapter 12
Paediatric emergencies

INTRODUCTION

Paediatric emergencies in the dental practice are fortunately very rare. However, if an emergency occurs, it is important to be able to respond quickly, effectively and safely. A sick child can deteriorate rapidly; it is most important to promptly recognise that a child is ill (ABCDE approach) and ensure appropriate help is sought. This may involve contacting the GP or calling 999 for an ambulance, depending on the situation. It is also important not to forget the child's parents or carer as they will usually be very upset and anxious.

If the child has a cardiopulmonary arrest in the dental practice, the adult resuscitation guidelines can be followed with just a few modifications to make them more suitable for a child. Cardiopulmonary arrest will most likely be secondary to a problem either with the airway or with breathing; hence the initial importance of oxygenation and ventilation.

To avoid misunderstanding, in this chapter, the terms 'child' and 'children' refer to both infants and children; when infants and children are specifically referred to, an infant can be defined as < 1 year and a child from 1 year to puberty.

The aim of this chapter is to provide a brief overview to the management of paediatric emergencies.

Learning outcomes

At the end of this chapter the reader will be able to:

- Outline the ABCDE assessment of a sick child
- Discuss the principles of paediatric resuscitation
- Describe the procedure for placing a child into the recovery position
- Discuss the management of foreign body airway obstruction

Age definitions for infants and children

Infant < 1 year

Child 1 year to puberty (use common sense)

(Biarent *et al.* 2005)

ABCDE ASSESSMENT OF A SICK CHILD

The ABCDE assessment of the sick patient has been described in detail in chapter 3. The same approach can be adopted when assessing a child, but with some modifications and additional considerations.

Whenever possible, keep the parent with the child when undertaking the assessment. Taking the child away from the parent may cause distress. If it is necessary to administer oxygen, ideally use a paediatric non-breathe mask (Figure 12.1); if the child does not tolerate this, asking the parent to hold an oxygen source near the child's face may be helpful.

Airway

Asking an infant or small child to talk in order to confirm airway patency will not be appropriate – look for other indicators of airway patency, e.g. vocalising and crying (Resuscitation Council (UK), 2006a).

Figure 12.1 Paediatric non-rebreathe mask.

PAEDIATRIC EMERGENCIES

Breathing

Normal respiratory rates are higher in children:

- < 1 year: 30–40 breaths per minute;
- 1–2 years: 26–34 breaths per minute;
- 2–5 years: 24–30 breaths per minute;
- 5–12 years 20–24 breaths per minute;
- > 12 years: 12–20 breaths per minute.
  (Resuscitation Council (UK), 2006a).

Look for chest recession or retractions (sternal, subcostal or intercostals) (indication of respiratory distress) (Resuscitation Council (UK), 2006a).

Circulation

Normal pulse rates are higher in children:

- 3 months–2 years: 100–180 beats per minute (when awake);
- 2–10 years: 60–140 beats per minute (when awake);
- > 10 years: 60–100 beats per minute (when awake).
  (Resuscitation Council (UK), 2006a).

Disability

Assess the child's interaction with his parents and surroundings. The parents will probably be able to advise whether this interaction is normal or not. Assess posture and tone: a seriously ill child becomes floppy.

Exposure

In any child who is unwell, look for the presence of tiny pink prick spots that can develop into purple bruising (purpuric rash) (Meningitis UK, 2009). This suggests bacterial meningitis. Try the tumbler test: press a glass tumbler against the rash – the rash will be visible through the glass and does not fade (Figure 12.2).

If exposing a child, take appropriate measures to minimise heat loss (particularly in infants) and respect the child's dignity (Resuscitation Council (UK), 2006a).

If possible record a core temperature, particularly if pyrexia is suspected.

Figure 12.2 Suspected bacterial meningitis: the tumbler test. Reproduced with kind permission from Meningitis UK, Registered Charity 1076774.

PRINCIPLES OF PAEDIATRIC RESUSCITATION

When undertaking paediatric resuscitation, the adult resuscitation guidelines described in chapter 9 can be followed, with some minor modifications. In this section, the modifications are listed, together with some background information, which the reader may find helpful.

Priorities

The two key priorities of resuscitation in children are:

- *Oxygenation and ventilation*: cardiorespiratory arrest in children is usually due to hypoxia (low oxygen levels in the blood);

- *Effective basic life support*: the most common cardiac arrhythmia is profound bradycardia (very slow heart rate) deteriorating to asystole (therefore the defibrillator is not usually required) (Resuscitation Council (UK), 2006a).

Therefore, the adult sequence of resuscitation described in chapter 9 would not be ideal if it was followed when resuscitation a child. However, a few minor modifications would make it suitable.

Modifications to the adult resuscitation guidelines

The procedure for resuscitation in children can follow the adult resuscitation guidelines; however four minor modifications will make the sequence more

PAEDIATRIC EMERGENCIES

suitable for use in children (Handley *et al.*, 2005; Resuscitation Council (UK), 2006b):

- Administer five initial ventilations before starting chest compressions.
- If alone, perform CPR for one minute before calling 999 for an ambulance.
- Compress the chest approximately one-third of its depth.
- Use two fingers when compressing the chest in an infant and in a child use one or two hands as needed to achieve the recommended depth of compression.

When to call 999 for an ambulance

As soon as it is confirmed that the child is not breathing normally, send someone to call 999 for an ambulance immediately. It is an emergency situation.

If the dental practitioner is alone (extremely rare), it is recommended to perform CPR for approximately one minute first before calling 999 (even if she has a mobile phone) (Resuscitation Council (UK), 2006b). The rationale for this is that prompt effective CPR may actually revive the child. It may be possible, after performing CPR for approximately a minute, to actually carry an infant or small child to the phone and continue CPR while calling 999 for an ambulance; this is recommended by some authorities (St John Ambulance *et al.*, 2006).

Airway management

The airway in an unconscious child can easily become obstructed by a combination of flexion of the neck, relaxation of the jaw, displacement of the tongue against the posterior wall of the pharynx and collapse of the hypopharynx: sometimes just opening the airway may revive the child (Jevon, 2009).

The airway can be opened by tilting the head and lifting the chin; this will help to open the airway and bring the tongue forward from the posterior wall of the pharynx (the tongue is most common cause of airway obstruction in an unconscious child; Jevon, 2003). The neutral position in an infant (Figure 12.3) and the sniffing the morning air position in a child (Figure 12.4) are recommended (Resuscitation Council (UK), 2006a).

Care should be taken not to press on the soft tissues under the chin as this may obstruct the airway, and blind finger sweeps are not recommended (Resuscitation Council (UK), 2006a). As in adults, if there is a history of trauma, the jaw thrust rather than head tilt/chin lift is recommended (Resuscitation Council (UK), 2006).

Figure 12.3 Opening the airway in an infant.

Figure 12.4 Opening the airway in a child.

An oropharyngeal airway can be used if there is difficulty achieving a patent airway, though particular care should be exercised if inserting one.

Ventilations

Once it is established that the child is not breathing normally, administer five initial ventilations (Figure 12.5) before, if needed, starting chest compressions at a ratio of 30 compressions to 2 ventilations (Resuscitation council (UK), 2006a). While performing these ventilations, send a colleague to call 999 for an ambulance.

Figure 12.5 Ventilations using a self-inflating bag.

Figure 12.6 Paediatric face masks.

PAEDIATRIC EMERGENCIES

It is recommended that a variety of child face masks (Figure 12.6) for attaching to a self-inflating bag should be immediately available in the dental practice (Resuscitation Council (UK), 2006). Ideally, a paediatric self-inflating bag should also be available, though in practice most dental practices will only have an adult bag available. An adult self-inflating bag can be used, though care should be taken to ensure that it is only squeezed enough to achieve visible chest rise. Regardless of the bag used, attach high flow oxygen (10 litres per minute) as soon as possible.

The use of a pocket mask is another option. The standard adult pocket mask can be used in an infant: position it upside down on the infant's face, ensuring that it covers the eye sockets as well as the nose and mouth (i.e. to achieve an

Figure 12.7 Using an adult pocket mask in an infant (upside down).

Figure 12.8 Paediatric pocket mask.

effective seal) (Figure 12.7). A paediatric pocket mask is also available (Figure 12.8).

If performing mouth to mouth resuscitation, apply a barrier face shield if one is available and if trained to use it. The principles of mouth to mouth ventilation in adults have been discussed in detail on pages 136–9. If performing mouth to mouth ventilation in an infant, place your mouth over the infant's nose and mouth to deliver the ventilations; in a child the technique used in adults can be followed. *Note:* just inflate sufficient air to achieve chest rise. After the initial five ventilations, perform 30 chest compressions to two ventilations as described above.

PAEDIATRIC EMERGENCIES

Chest compressions

The principles of performing chest compressions in children are the same as in adults, with two minor modifications:

- Compress the chest approximately one-third of its depth.
- Use two fingers when compressing the chest in an infant and in a child use one or two hands as needed to achieve the recommended depth of compression.

Chest compressions in an infant

- Deliver five initial ventilations.
- Place the tips of two fingers in the centre of the chest (taking care not to press on the lower tip of the sternum, the ribs or the abdomen) (Figure 12.9).
- Compress the chest vertically down about one third of its depth and then release the pressure to allow the chest to fully re-expand (without losing contact with the chest) (St John Ambulance et al., 2006). Not allowing the chest to fully re-expand will hinder venous return to the heart and reduce the blood flow to the vital organs (Jevon, 2003).
- Compress the chest at a rate of 100 per minute with a ratio of 30 compressions to two ventilations (Handley et al., 2005).
- If alone, after performing CPR for approximately one minute, call 999 for an ambulance.

Figure 12.9 Chest compressions in an infant.

Chest compressions in a child

- Deliver five initial ventilations.

- Place the heal of one hand in the centre of the chest (taking care not to press on the lower tip of the sternum, the ribs or the abdomen) (Figure 12.10a). In an older child or if struggling to achieve the recommended compression depth, use the two-handed technique (Figure 12.10b).

- Compress the chest vertically down about one third of its depth and then release the pressure to allow the chest to fully re-expand (without losing contact with the chest) (St John Ambulance *et al.*, 2006).

- Compress the chest at a rate of 100 per minute with a ratio of 30 compressions to two ventilations (Handley *et al.*, 2005).

- If working alone, after performing CPR for approximately one minute, call 999 for an ambulance.

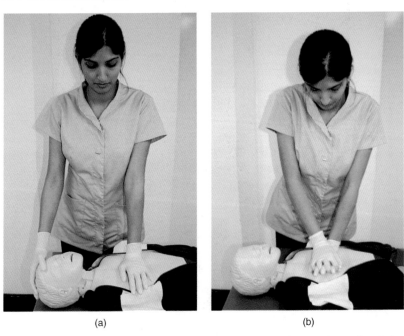

(a)   (b)

Figure 12.10 Chest compressions in a child: (a) one handed technique; (b) two handed technique.

The use of automated external defibrillators in children

Most cardiac arrests in children are secondary to a life-threatening airway or breathing problem; as discussed above, the initial priorities in paediatric

Figure 12.11 Paediatric AED pads.

resuscitation are to open and clear the airway and ventilate with high concentration oxygen; defibrillation is rarely indicated.

However, very occasionally the primary cause of a paediatric cardiorespiratory arrest will be ventricular fibrillation (see page 151), a shockable rhythm. Automated external defibrillators (AEDs) have been used successfully in children (Gurnett & Atkins, 2000; Konig *et al.*, 2005). Most AED manufacturers now supply paediatric pads (Figure 12.11) or programmes which will usually limit the voltage output of the AED to 50–75 J (Jorgenson *et al.*, 2002); these devices are recommended for children aged between 1 and 8 years (Berg *et al.*, 2004). However, if one of these devices is not available, it is recommended to use an unmodified adult AED in children over 1 year of age (Berg *et al.*, 2005).

The use of AEDs in adults has been described in detail in chapter 11. If using an AED in a child, it is important to follow the manufacturer's recommendations, particularly if using specifically designed paediatric pads or programme.

PLACING A CHILD INTO THE RECOVERY POSITION

If an infant or child is unconscious, but breathing normally, she should be placed into the recovery position; this will help to prevent the tongue falling back and obstructing the airway and will reduce the risk of inhalation of stomach contents (Resuscitation Council (UK), 2006).

There are several recovery positions currently advocated, but no single one can be endorsed. However, there are some important key principles that need to be followed when placing an infant or child in the recovery position (Biarent *et al.*, 2005):

- *Lateral position*: as far as possible, the true lateral position should be adopted, with the mouth dependent to allow free drainage of fluid.

- *Stability*: the position used should be stable; in an infant a rolled-up cushion or blanket (or similar) placed behind the back may be necessary to maintain the position.

- *Ease of monitoring*: it should be possible to easily observe (and access) the airway and monitor breathing.

- *Ease of repositioning*: it should be easy to reposition the child or roll her back into the supine position.

- *Avoidance of pressure on the chest*: the position should not result in pressure being applied to the chest that impairs breathing.

The recovery position in adults described on pages 85–9 can be used in children, though some modification may be required.

MANAGEMENT OF FOREIGN BODY AIRWAY OBSTRUCTION

Foreign body airway obstruction is a life-threatening emergency, often characterised by a sudden inability to talk, maximal respiratory effort, development of cyanosis and clutching of the neck (Jevon, 2003). There may be a history of the child eating a sweet or playing with a small object.

Back slaps, chest thrusts and abdominal thrusts can all help expel a foreign body from the airway (Biarent *et al.*, 2005); however, in 50% of choking episodes, more than one technique will be required to relieve the obstruction (Redding, 1979).

Blind finger sweeps

In all situations it would be helpful to remove any obvious foreign body from the mouth, but blind finger sweeps are not recommended as they could further impact the foreign body (Jevon, 2003) and may actually cause pharyngeal trauma.

Resuscitation Council (UK) choking guidelines

The Resuscitation Council (UK) adult choking guidelines (see pages 145–8) are also suitable for use in children over 1 year of age. They can also be followed for an infant, but with a slight modification, i.e. chest thrusts instead of abdominal thrusts (Biarent *et al.*, 2005).

Effective and ineffective cough

In a conscious child the treatment is determined by whether he has an effective cough or not (Biarent *et al.*, 2005):

- *Effective cough*: crying or a verbal response to questions, loud cough, ability to breathe before coughing and fully responsive;
- *Ineffective cough*: inability to vocalise, quiet or silent cough, inability to breathe, cyanosis and decreasing level of consciousness.

Treatment of an infant with foreign body airway obstruction

If the infant has foreign body airway obstruction, but has an effective cough, encourage him to cough. If the infant has (or is developing) an ineffective cough, but is still conscious (Biarent *et al.*, 2005; Jevon, 2003):

1. Call out for help.

2. Support the infant in a prone position, e.g. resting on your forearm or across your lap, ensuring that the head is lower than the chest (gravity will assist removal of the foreign body) and the head is well supported.

3. Deliver up to five sharp blows between the shoulder blades using the heel of the hand (Figure 12.12). If the back slaps fail to dislodge the foreign body, proceed to chest thrusts.

4. Turn the infant into a supine position, ensuring again that the head is lower than the chest.

5. Deliver up to five chest thrusts to the sternum (similar to chest compressions, but more vigorous, sharper and slower, at a rate of one every 3 seconds) (Jevon, 2003).

6. Recheck the mouth and carefully remove any visible foreign body.

7. If the airway remains obstructed, repeat the above steps as necessary.

Figure 12.12 Treatment of FBAO in an infant: back blows.

If the infant becomes unconscious, if not already, ask a colleague to call 999 for an ambulance and follow the resuscitation protocols, i.e. open and clear the airway, attempt to deliver five ventilations before starting chest compressions (ratio 30:2 as above).

Abdominal thrusts are NOT recommended in infants (Resuscitation Council (UK), 2006)

Treatment of a child with foreign body airway obstruction

This is the same as for adults, as described on pages 145–8, and therefore only a brief description is required here. If the child has an ineffective cough, administer back blows (Figure 12.13); if these fail to dislodge the foreign body, proceed to abdominal thrusts.

Figure 12.13 Treatment of FBAO in a child: back blows.

CONCLUSION

Paediatric emergencies in the dental practice are rare. If one occurs, it is important to be able to respond quickly, effectively and safely. In this chapter an overview has been provided of the management of paediatric emergencies. The ABCDE assessment of a sick child has been outlined and the principles of paediatric resuscitation have been discussed. The procedure for placing a child into the recovery position and the management of foreign body airway obstruction have been described.

REFERENCES

Berg R, Chapman F, Berg M *et al.* (2004) Attenuated adult biphasic shocks compared with weight-based monophasic shocks in a swine model or prolonged pediatric ventricular fibrillation. *Resuscitation*; 61:189–197.

Berg R, Samson R, Berg M *et al.* (2005) Better outcome after paediatric defibrillation dosage than adult dosage in a swine model of pediatric ventricular fibrillation. *J Am Coll Cardiol*; 45:786–789.

PAEDIATRIC EMERGENCIES

Biarent D, Bingham R, Richmond S *et al.* (2005) European Resuscitation Council Guidelines for Resuscitation 2005: Section 6. Paediatric life support. *Resuscitation* 67S1, S97–S133.

Gurnett C, Atkins D (2000) Successful use of a biphasic waveform automated external defibrillator in a high-risk child. *American Journal of Cardiology*; 86:1051–1053.

Handley A, Koster R, Monsieurs K *et al.* (2005) Adult basic life support and use of automated external defibrillators. *Resuscitation*; 67: Suppl. S7–23.

Jevon P (2003) *Paediatric Advanced Life Support*. Elsevier, Edinburgh.

Jevon P (2009) *Advanced Cardiac Life Support*, 2nd edn. Wiley-Blackwell, Oxford.

Jorgenson D, Morgan C, Snyder D *et al.* (2002) Energy attenuator for pediatric application of an automated external defibrillator. *Critical Care Medicine*; 30:S145–S147.

Konig B, Benger J, Goldsworthy L (2005) Automated external defibrillation in a 6-year-old. *Archives of Disease in Childhood*; 90:310–311.

Meningitis UK (2009) www.meningitisuk.org (accessed 7 March 2009).

Redding J (1979) The choking controversy: critique of evidence of the Heimlich maneuver. *Critical Care Medicine*; 7:475–479.

Resuscitation Council (UK) (2006a) *Paediatric Immediate Life Support*, 1st edn. Resuscitation Council (UK), London.

Resuscitation Council (UK) (2006b) *Medical emergencies and resuscitation standards for clinical practice and training for dental practitioners and dental care professionals in general dental practice*. Resuscitation Council (UK), London.

St John Ambulance, St Andrew's Ambulance, British Red Cross (2006) *First Aid Manual*, 9th edn. Dorling Kindersley, London.

PAEDIATRIC EMERGENCIES

Chapter 13

Professional and legal issues

Richard Griffith

INTRODUCTION

Law and ethics are now fundamental to the practice of dentistry and underpin your relationship with the profession and with your patients. The law informs dentistry at every stage and it is essential that dental professionals understand and are able to critically reflect on the legal issues relevant to practice. This is particularly true in emergency situations when an appropriate and timely response is required.

When dental professionals treat patients they undertake a duty of care towards those persons not to harm them in accordance with the law of negligence. Where dental professionals provide treatment to a patient for a fee then that treatment will be regulated under the laws of contract with the patient able to sue if the contract is not fulfilled. Dental professionals' right to touch a patient will be based on the law of consent and the informed and freely given permission of the patient will be a prerequisite to any lawful treatment. The legal principles of confidentiality and negligence regulate the relationship between the dental professional and the patient while they are in the professional's care.

The standards of the profession and its regulatory body, the General Dental Council, are derived from fundamental human rights principles. These principles largely underpin the law relating to healthcare and the standards of conduct and performance required of dental professionals by the General Dental Council's *Standards for Dental Professionals* (2005a).

LEARNING OUTCOMES

At the end of this chapter the reader will be able to:

- Discuss the scope of a dental professional's accountability
- Outline the legal requirements for consent and acting in a patient's best interests
- State the extent of the duty of confidence owed to patients by dental professionals
- Explain the principles of patient safety

THE SCOPE OF A DENTAL PROFESSIONAL'S ACCOUNTABILITY

A registered dental professional is legally and professionally accountable for his or her actions, irrespective of whether they are following the instruction of another or using their own initiative. Healthcare litigation is increasing and patients are increasingly prepared to assert their legal rights. It perhaps little wonder therefore that the General Dental Council insist that dental professionals are able to practise in accordance with an ethical and legal framework which ensures the primacy of patient and client interest (General Dental Council, 2005a,b).

A thorough and critical appreciation of the legal and professional issues affecting dental practice is essential if you are to develop the professional awareness necessary to satisfy the General Dental Council that you are an accountable practitioner, competent to practise as a registered dental professional (see Table 13.1).

Table 13.1 Advantages of legal awareness for the dental professional

The legally aware dental professional:

- Realises that many aspects of daily life are governed by law
  Most aspects of life are regulated by law. Legal awareness helps the dental professional appreciate the importance of the legal framework which supports the structure of society. It also allows the dental professional to appreciate that personal and social problems may have a legal dimension.
- Knowingly acts in accordance with legal principles
  Many parts of the law are necessarily complex and difficult to understand. However, the underlying principles are quite simple. These affect everyone on a day-to-day basis and therefore an understanding of them is important. Indeed, ignorance of the law can bring very serious consequences.
- Understands the key elements of the legal system
  Knowledge of the law is of limited value without understanding the various ways in which the legal system works to enforce the law.
  It is important to understand the role of those agencies which have powers to enforce the law and the mechanisms by which the dental professional can seek legal help and advice.
- Knows when and where to seek appropriate advice
  The law is vast and constantly changing. The dental professional needs to develop a sense of:
  a) when the law can help or hinder
  b) what can be found out and where
  c) when to should seek expert help and
  d) how to get the appropriate help or advice.
- Understands the nature of law

Even though many day-to-day situations have a legal dimension, there are some problems which the law can do little about, even when in theory this should not be the case.

Defining accountability

In their seminal work on the subject, Lewis and Batey (1982) defined accountability as 'the fulfilment of a formal obligation to disclose to reverent others the purposes, principles, procedures, relationships, results, income and expenditures for which one has authority.'

An analysis of Lewis and Batey's definition reveals the fundamental nature of accountability. The 'fulfilment of a formal obligation' suggests that accountability has its basis in law. That is, there is a formal or legal relationship between the practitioner and higher authorities (the 'reverent others') that are entitled to hold the dental professional to account. The extent of the scrutiny is illustrated by the inclusion of 'the purposes, principles, procedures, relationships, results, income and expenditures for which one has authority' in the definition. Put more concisely, to be accountable is to be answerable for the acts and omissions within your practice.

This is the approach adopted by the General Dental Council (2005a), the profession's regulatory body, who state in *Standards for Dental Professionals* that:

'You have a professional responsibility to be prepared to justify your actions, and we may ask you to do so. You must be willing and able to show that you are aware of this booklet; and you have followed the principles it explains.

'If you cannot give a satisfactory account of your behaviour or practice in line with the principles explained in this booklet, your registration will be at risk.'

Accountability may be defined as being answerable for personal acts or omissions to a higher authority with whom the dental professional has a legal relationship.

Exercising accountability

A common misconception about accountability is that a dentist has some choice over what they are accountable for. Meeting their professional responsibility is often expressed as exercising accountability.

While it is true to say that the General Dental Council sets out the standard of conduct required of dental professionals, accountability cannot be exercised as this would require the practitioner to have control over what they were accountable for. It suggests that dentists can pick and choose whether they wish to be accountable for this action or that patient. This cannot be the case as the purpose of accountability is to protect the public and offer redress to those who have been harmed by dental professionals' acts or omissions. Dental professionals are answerable through the law to a number of higher authorities

Table 13.2 Functions of accountability

Protective function – the purpose of accountability is to protect the public from the acts or omissions of dental professionals that might cause harm

Deterrent function – The threat of sanction available to the higher authorities against registered practitioners is seen as protecting the public by deterring acts or omissions that might cause harm

Regulatory function – By making the dental professional accountable to a range of higher authorities the law regulates their behaviour and allows action to be taken to protect the public should they breach the regulatory framework

Educative function – Accountability has an educative function in that those found liable have their cases heard in public with a view to reassuring society that only the highest standards of practice will be tolerated. Other practitioners will learn from such cases and refrain from acting in a similar manner

and it is these higher authorities, not the professionals themselves, who decide if they are to be held to account.

Accountability has four functions as set out in Table 13.2.

Accountable to whom?

Dental professionals owe a formal obligation to answer for their practice to a range of higher authorities. These have a legal relationship with you that enable them to demand that you justify your practice. If you fail to satisfy those requirements, sanctions may be applied against you.

In order to provide maximum protection to the public four areas of law are drawn together and can individually or collectively hold you to account. Figure 13.1 depicts to whom you are accountable as a dental professional and the legal basis of that relationship.

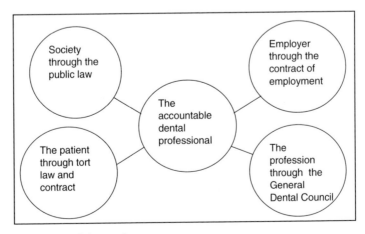

Figure 13.1 Accountability to whom.

PROFESSIONAL AND LEGAL ISSUES

Accountability to society

Dental professionals are subject to the same laws as any other member of society. There is nothing about the status of a dentist that exempts them from these laws. If a dentist is suspected of committing a crime during the course of their practice or otherwise they can be called to account.

Accountability to society is achieved through the public law. Many of these laws are derived from Acts of Parliament such as the Road Traffic Act 1988, the Theft Act 1968 or the Offences Against the Person Act 1861. Such Acts are known as public general acts and it is entirely possible to breach them in the course of your practice. For example, a dentist claimed payments for the same patients from two neighbouring health authorities. Investigators uncovered false addresses and a £73,000 fraud. The dentist was convicted and jailed for 12 months (Hope, 1994).

The treatment a dental professional provides to their patient often requires interventions that are personal and intimate in nature. The public law demands that such interventions are only carried out when it is convincingly shown to be medically necessary and by staff who are properly qualified (*R* v *Tabassum* [2000]). Where this occurs the dentist's actions stand outside the criminal law (*Airedale NHS Trust* v *Bland* [1993]). However, the acts of the dental professional will lose their immunity if the necessity cannot be made out or the treatment proceeds without either the consent of a capable patient or the best interests of an incapable patient. For example, a dental practitioner who repeatedly touched a female patient in unnecessary intimate examinations was sentenced to 9 months imprisonment for indecent assault that the judge described as a gross breach of trust (*Yorkshire Evening Post*, 2008).

The public law seeks to protect patients through the regulation of practice and the environment of care. The National Health Service Litigation Authority (2007) estimates that some £500 million is paid annually by the health service in compensation claims and fines for breaching health and safety laws. The cost in human terms can also be high. Mistakes and errors can compromise safety to the point where lives are put at risk and, sadly, fatalities do occur.

To prevent the avoidable loss of life and minimise the days lost to absence an employer has a legal duty to comply with the requirements relating to health and safety at work. The Health and Safety at Work etc. Act 1974 is the basis of health and safety law in the United Kingdom and it sets out general duties which:

- employers have towards employees and members of the public using their service; and

- employees have to themselves and to each other.

Breaching or failing to comply with these duties are criminal offences.

The employer's general duty is set out in section 2 of the Health and Safety at Work etc. Act 1974 and states that an employer has a duty to ensure *so far as is reasonably practicable*, the health, safety and welfare at work of employees and any others who may be affected by the undertaking.

The legal standard imposed by the 1974 Act is *reasonably practicable* or *so far as is reasonably practicable*. The standard implies a weighing up of the risk against the cost in terms of time, money or trouble of preventing or controlling the risk.

The duty of employees at work is set out in section 7 of the Health and Safety at Work etc. Act 1974 that states that:

'It shall be the duty of every employee whilst at work:

- To take reasonable care of their own health and safety and of any other person who may be affected by their acts or omissions; and

- To co-operate with their employer so far as is necessary to enable that employer to meet their requirements with regards to any statutory provisions.'

As well as a duty under the Health and Safety at Work etc. Act 1974 a dental professional is also under a professional duty to act to identify and minimise the risk to patients and clients (General Dental Council 2005a).

The General Dental Council (2005a) has acknowledged that medical emergencies can occur at any time so all members of staff must know their role in the event of a medical emergency. It is essential therefore that dental professionals and their staff are suitably trained in dealing with emergencies and practise together regularly in simulated emergency situations to maintain their competence. This includes where to locate and use an automated external defibrillator.

A dental professional who raises an issue of health and safety with an employer either directly or through a union is entitled to protection from dismissal and victimisation under the Public Interest Disclosure Act 1998. Under the Act each NHS employer has a duty to establish a procedure for employees to raise concerns where:

- a criminal offence has been, is being or is likely to be committed; or

- the health or safety of an individual has been, is being or is likely to be endangered.

It is essential that employers and staff work together to ensure effective implementation of health and safety measures. This joint approach helps to promote and raise awareness among employers and staff, thereby creating a positive safety culture.

PROFESSIONAL AND LEGAL ISSUES

Workplace risk assessments

A risk assessment is the identification of hazards present in the workplace and an estimate of the risk associated with performing the task. A hazard is something that has the potential to cause harm and a risk is the likelihood of that hazard causing an accident or incident.

There is a legal duty to perform risk assessments under the provisions of the Management of Health and Safety at Work Regulations 1999.

Once a hazard has been identified the likelihood of the risk occurring and the severity of the harm must be considered. The law requires that risks should be reduced *so far as is reasonably practicable*. That means that the degree of risk should be balanced against the time, trouble, cost and physical difficulty of taking measures to avoid it.

On identifying a risk, steps must be taken to minimise it by:

- Elimination of the hazard at source, if this is not possible then the hazard must be reduced;

- If the hazard has to be reduced then action must be taken to control the risk by introducing workplace precautions such as alarms, training and information, safety cabinets, ventilation systems, etc;

- Once workplace precautions have been introduced then a system to monitor compliance with those precautions must be put in place.

Medicines

Modern dental practice often requires the use of medicines in the treatment of patients. While medicines are used for their therapeutic benefits they can and do cause adverse effects in some patients. In *Forman v Saroya* [1992] a woman contracted hepatitis as a result of a reaction to halothane anaesthetic administered by her dentist. The dentist ought to have known of her susceptibility because she had suffered a similar reaction when he had given it on a previous occasion. The patient experienced severe abdominal pains soon after the halothane anaesthetic was administered and began to vomit, then suffered lethargy and loss of appetite. These symptoms persisted for just over two weeks and required a period in hospital. The dentist was found negligent.

The principal statutory framework for the regulation of medicines is the Medicines Act 1968. The Act regulates the licensing, supply and administration of medicines. The Secretary of State for Health has a duty under s.58A Medicines Act 1968 to place on prescription only medicines that represent a danger to the patient if their use is not supervised by an appropriate practitioner. Therefore, prescription-only medicines may only be administered by or in accordance with the directions of an appropriate practitioner (Medicines Act 1968, s.58(2)(b)).

Appropriate practitioners include registered dentists who have their own formulary of medicines from which they are authorised to prescribe (Medicines Act 1968, s.58(1)). Other dental professionals are not appropriate practitioners and generally must only administer medicines in accordance with the directions issued by an appropriate practitioner.

A degree of flexibility over the supply and administration of prescription-only medicines to patients has been provided by the introduction of Patient Group Directions which is a written instruction for the supply or administration of a licensed medicine in an identified clinical situation where the patient may not be individually identified before presenting for treatment.

A Patient Group Direction is drawn up locally by doctors, pharmacists and other health professionals and must meet the legal criteria set out in the Prescription Only Medicines (Human Use) Amendment Order 2000. Patient Group Directions can only be used by registered healthcare professionals acting as named individuals, and a list of individuals named as competent to supply and administer medicines under the direction must be included.

Articles 12B, 12C and 12E of the Prescription Only Medicines (Human Use) Order 1997 exempt registered health professionals from the need to obtain a prescription to supply a prescription-only medicine if they act according to a valid Patient Group Direction.

A Patient Specific Direction is a written instruction for prescription-only medicines to be supplied for administering to a named patient without a prescription. An example would be an instruction by a dentist to supply and administer a medicine in the surgery such as an antibiotic.

The Prescription Only Medicines (Human Use) Order 1997 authorises the use of Patient Specific Directions. Article 12 of the order allows any appropriate practitioner (including dentists) to authorise the supply of a prescription-only medicine for the purpose of being administered to a specific person. To be valid the Patient Specific Direction must:

- be in writing;

- relate to the particular person to whom the medicine is to be administered; and

- be issued by a dentist.

Exemption in an emergency

In an emergency certain prescription-only medicines may be supplied and administered without prescription. The Prescription Only Medicines (Human Use) Order 1997, article 7 allows for the parenteral administration of prescription-only medicines including adrenaline and hydrocortisone injection for the purpose of saving life in an emergency and there is no specific restriction on who is entitled to administer these medicines.

Accountability to the patient

As well as being accountable to society in general, dental professionals are also accountable to the individual patients in their care. The tort or civil law system allows a patient to sue for compensation if they believe that harm has been caused through carelessness. Liability for carelessness is given its legal expression in the law relating to negligence.

Negligence is a civil wrong and best defined as actionable harm. That is, a person sues for compensation because they have been harmed by the carelessness of another person.

Negligence in the healthcare setting has developed under the common law by judges setting rules through decided cases. In certain circumstances, called duty situations, the nature of the relationship between people gives rise to a duty of care. For example, a manufacturer owes a duty to the consumer of his product (*Donoghue* v *Stevenson* [1932]) and one road user owes a duty of care to the other road users in his vicinity (*Rouse* v *Squires* [1973]). Similarly the dentist–patient relationship gives rise to a duty of care (*Kent* v *Griffiths* [2001]). Dentists owe their patients a duty of care and are accountable to the patient if they cause harm by breaching that duty.

In civil law dental professionals are expected to meet the standard of care set by reference to *Bolam* v *Friern HMC* [1957]. Known as the Bolam test, it requires that dental professionals meet the standard of the ordinary skilled person exercising and professing to have that special skill or art (*Gold* v *Haringey HA* [1998]).

Case law demonstrates that the standard covers the whole of the professional relationship with the patient and includes direct care (*Bayliss* v *Blagg & another* (1954)), advice giving and record-keeping (*Greenfield* v *Irwin (A Firm)* [2001]), even the standard of handwriting (*Prendergast* v *Sam and Dee* [1989]). If the dental professional's actions were in keeping with a respected body of professional opinion then practice will not have fallen below the standard required in law and there will be no liability in negligence (*Bolam* v *Friern HMC* [1957]). This will be the case even if there were different ways of performing a task. A judge cannot find negligence just because he prefers one professional's view over another (*Maynard* v *West Midlands RHA* [1984]).

However, in *Bolitho* v *City & Hackney HA* [1997] the House of Lords held that any expert evidence used to support a dentist's actions must stand up to logical analysis. That is, the existence of a common practice does not necessarily mean that it is not negligent. A defendant will not be exonerated because others too are negligent or because common professional practice is slack.

The duty of care to the patient also requires dental professionals to keep their knowledge up to date throughout their career (*Roe* v *Ministry of Health* [1954]).

Emergencies

Dental professionals continue to owe their patient a duty of care in an emergency situation. They are expected to be able to respond effectively to the common emergencies that might arise in dental surgeries. They are expected to ensure that their practice is up to date and evidence based (*Reynolds* v *North Tyneside Health Authority* [2002]).

In relation to treatment decisions taken in an emergency, a dental professional will not be found negligent simply because the reasonably competent dentist would have made a different decision, given more time and information.

In *Wilson* v *Swanson* (1956), the Supreme Court of Canada held that there was no negligence when a surgeon had to make an immediate decision whether to operate during an emergency, when the operation was subsequently found to have been unnecessary.

Moreover, the skill required in the execution of treatment may be somewhat lower because an emergency may overburden the available resources, and, if a dental professional is forced by circumstances to do too many things at once, the fact that he or she does one of them incorrectly would not lightly be taken as negligence.

Carelessness as a crime

Although legal proceedings for carelessness are usually instigated at civil law, it is possible to face criminal prosecution where gross negligence has occurred. In *R* v *Misra & Srivasta* [2004] the Court of Appeal stated that a health professional would be told that grossly negligent treatment which exposed a patient to the risk of death, and caused it, would constitute manslaughter. In this case two doctors refused to call for timely assistance when informed by nurses that a patient was severely ill. The patient died of toxic shock and the doctors were given 14-month suspended jail terms.

Death of a patient in the dental surgery

Where a patient dies in a dental surgery it will likely be an unnatural or sudden death. Such deaths fall into the category that must be reported to the coroner. This includes deaths where:

- the cause of death is unknown;
- the deceased was not seen by the certifying doctor either after death or within the 14 days before death;
- the death was violent or unnatural or suspicious;
- the death may be due to an accident (whenever it occurred);

- the death may be due to self-neglect or neglect by others;
- the death may be due to an industrial disease or related to the deceased's employment;
- the death may be due to an abortion;
- the death occurred during an operation or before recovery from the effects of an anaesthetic;
- the death may be a suicide;
- the death occurred during or shortly after detention in police or prison custody.

It will therefore be necessary to inform the police as well as the emergency medical services of the death. The scene of the death will need to be preserved including the equipment and medicines used so that they can be noted by the police or coroner's officer. Staff involved in the incident should remain available to give a statement for use by the coroner at the inquest.

Accountability to the employer

An employed dental professional is accountable to their employer through the contract of employment. The contract sets out the terms and conditions of employment and the standard of work expected of the employee (Rideout, 1983). Many of these terms are written in the contract such as salary, holiday entitlement, hours of work, etc. and are known as express contract terms.

In addition many conditions that regulate the relationship between employer and employee are not expressly written into the contract but are there by virtue of decided cases or employment-related legislation. These are known as implied contract terms and include a warranty from the employee to the employer that they will carry out their duties with due care and diligence (*Harmer* v *Cornelius* (1858)).

Employers are liable for any compensation payable as a result of a civil wrong committed by an employee during the course of their employment, through vicarious liability. Employers will wish to minimise that liability and are entitled under contract law to hold their employees to account through reasonable disciplinary procedures.

For dental professionals, their employer is the most likely authority to hold them to account as a patient with a grievance is more likely to complain to the employer than take legal action. In addition, employment law allows a lower burden of proof when deciding whether an employee is guilty of misconduct.

Unlike criminal law, where the prosecution must prove a case beyond reasonable doubt, or civil law, where a person must show on the balance of probability that a tort was committed against them, employment law only requires that an employer hold an honest and genuine belief that the employee is guilty of misconduct based on the outcome of a reasonable investigation (*British Home Stores Ltd* v *Burchell* [1980]).

Accountability to the profession

Dental professionals are accountable to the profession through the provisions of the Dentists Act 1984 and Health Act 1999, section 60.

The General Dental Council's role is to protect the public by establishing standards of education, training, conduct and performance for dental professionals including all dentists, dental nurses, dental technicians, dental hygienists, dental therapists, clinical dental technicians and orthodontic therapists who must be registered with the council in order to practise.

The General Dental Council is concerned with protecting the public, not dealing with local issues such as a breach of employment contract. Only where the conduct or performance of a dental professional gives rise to concern for public safety will the General Dental Council become involved.

Fitness to practise is the term now used by the General Dental Council to describe a registrant's suitability to be on the register without restrictions. The General Dental Council has the power to hold a registered dental practitioner to account if it is alleged that their fitness to practise is impaired.

The standards by which practitioners are judged and the General Dental Council considers the public are entitled to expect are set out in the *Standards for Dental Professionals* (General Dental Council 2005a). Practitioners who appear before the General Dental Council's fitness to practise panels are held to account against those standards. The standard of conduct and competence expected by the General Dental Council is that of the average practitioner, not the highest possible level of practice. This approach is similar to that adopted by the civil law when judging a skilled practitioner under the Bolam test to determine whether liability in negligence has arisen.

The key difference between negligence law and professional accountability though is that no action in negligence can occur without harm to the patient. However, a breach of the code can occur and a practitioner be held to account even though there has been no harm to a patient.

Strengthening public confidence in the General Dental Council

The General Dental Council is itself regulated by the Council for the Regulation of Healthcare Professionals which oversees the disciplinary decisions of the main bodies of the healthcare professions. It has the power under section 29 of the National Health Service Reform and Health Care Professions Act 2002 to seek a judicial review of a disciplinary decision of a healthcare regulatory body where it considers that decision to be unduly lenient. For example, in *Council for the Regulation of Healthcare Professionals* v *General Dental Council* [2005] the General Dental Council suspended the licence of a dentist to practise for 12 months after he was sentenced to a 3-year community punishment for offences under the Protection of Children Act 1978. The Council for the Regulation of Healthcare Professionals argued that the General Dental Council's sanction in the case was unduly lenient. The court held that a suspension for 12 months was unduly lenient given the serious nature of the offences. The court ordered that in this case removal from the register was the only appropriate penalty.

It can be seen that you are accountable to the profession through the provisions of the Dentist Act 1984 as amended by the Health Act 1999 that empower the General Dental Council to maintain a professional register of dental care practitioners and to determine the standards of education and training necessary to enter the register and to establish standards for practice in order to remain on the register. The standards expected of a registered practitioner are set out in *Standards for Dental Professionals* (General Dental Council 2005a).

LEGAL REQUIREMENTS FOR CONSENT AND ACTING IN A PATIENT'S BEST INTERESTS

A key requirement of the *Standards for Dental Professionals* concerns respect for patient dignity and choice. Dental professionals are required to:

'Recognise and promote patients' responsibility for making decisions about their bodies, their priorities and their care, making sure you do not take any steps without patients' consent.' (General Dental Council 2005b at point 2)

Dental professionals need to touch their patients in order to examine or administer treatment or dental care (*F* v *West Berkshire HA* [1990]). The right to touch an individual is limited in law and there is an initial presumption that it must not occur without consent.

The right to self determination

The law recognises that adults have a right to determine what will be done to their bodies (*Schloendroff* v *Society of New York Hospitals* (1914)). Touching a person without consent will amount to a trespass to the person or, rarely, a criminal assault. Bodily integrity is held in very high regard by the law. Unlike other civil wrongs, such as negligence, that requires harm, any unlawful touching is actionable even if done with the best of motives.

Free choice allows patients to refuse treatment even where this is not in their best interests or might lead to serious health consequences (*Re MB (Caesarean Section)* [1997]). As the right to self determination is held in such high regard it is essential that dental professionals obtain a valid consent from their patients before proceeding with treatment.

Elements of a valid consent

To be a valid defence to a claim of trespass, consent needs to be full, free and reasonably informed.

Full consent

When obtaining consent a patient must agree to all the treatment being proposed (*Williamson* v *East London & City HA* [1998]). Dental professionals must take care to explain all the treatment or touching that will occur when obtaining consent from a patient and ensure that additional treatment or touching is subject to further consent.

Free consent

Consent is an expression of autonomy and must be the free choice of the individual. It cannot be obtained by undue influence (*Re T* [1992]). This does not mean that a dental professional cannot influence a patient's decision. Indeed part of your role is to explain the benefits of treatment to patients in order to obtain consent.

In law to be undue influence the action must erode the free will of the patient (*Re U* [2002]). It must be so forceful that the patient excludes all other considerations when making their choice. Undue influence may also be brought to bear by family members. Dental professionals must be certain that the choice being made is that of the patient and not the outside influence of family members (*Re T (Adult: Refusal of Treatment)* [1992]).

Reasonably informed consent

In order to make a free choice a person needs to have sufficient information to inform that choice. For consent to be real, dental professionals are required to explain in general terms what the procedure entails. If a patient can show that the procedure was not explained in broad terms then the consent would be vitiated and liability in trespass would result (*Chatterton* v *Gerson* [1981]).

As well as a general explanation of the procedure there is also a duty to explain the risks inherent in the procedure. Failing to meet this legal duty will give rise to an action in negligence if the patient was subsequently harmed (*Sidaway* v *Bethlem Royal Hospital* [1985]).

It can be seen that taking consent is more that accepting the patient's permission. To be a valid consent the decision must be full, free and reasonably informed.

Fraudulent consent

Consent to examination or treatment obtained by fraud will be invalid (*Chatterton* v *Gerson* [1981]). Such a situation would arise where a dental professional obtained consent for unnecessary treatment from patients.

In *Appleton* v *Garrett* [1997] a registered dentist was sued in negligence and trespass for gross overtreatment of patients. The court found that the dentist deliberately embarked on treatment that was unnecessary while deliberately misleading patients as to its necessity because he knew that otherwise they would not have consented to the treatment. The consent was obtained by fraud and was not real and informed consent.

Obtaining consent

Dental professionals may obtain consent in two ways. First, a patient may express their consent. That is, a patient makes known their willingness to be touched. Express consent can be written or oral.

Written consent is usually obtained where a procedure is invasive or perceived as carrying a material risk. A consent form provides a degree of evidential certainty that the patient agreed to treatment. It should not be relied on too heavily, however. Lord Donaldson in *Re T* [1982] pointed out that a consent form was only as useful as the understanding of the person signing it. When obtaining consent, whether in writing or orally, it is essential that an explanation of treatment and other material facts must be recorded in the patient's file to corroborate the consent.

The second form of consent is an implied consent. This is permission implied through the actions of the patient. A patient opening their mouth when the dental professional asks to examine their teeth is a typical example of an implied consent, as permission to proceed is implied from the action of the patient in response to a request to carry out an examination. It does not mean that agreeing to come to the hospital or surgery implies that a patient agrees to all treatment. Every episode of treatment must be subject to a valid consent.

Consent is a continuous process and may be withdrawn at any time. A withdrawal of consent is as indistinguishable as an initial refusal to consent (*Ciarlariello* v *Schacter* [1991]). Dental professionals must accept that if a patient changes their mind and refuses to continue with treatment then treatment must cease or trespass will occur.

PROFESSIONAL AND LEGAL ISSUES

Capacity and self determination

Capacity in law is the ability to understand and make a balanced decision and is the key to autonomy (*Re T (Adult: Refusal of Treatment)* [1992]). If a person has capacity, dental professionals are bound by their decision. If not, the Mental Capacity Act 2005 can allow another person to make that decision or require the dental professional to determine if the treatment is in their patient's best interests.

Mental Capacity Act 2005

The Mental Capacity Act 2005 sets out a framework for acting for and making decisions on behalf of people aged 16 years and over who lack the mental capacity to make decisions for themselves.

The statutory principles

To underline the Act's fundamental concepts, section 1 establishes a number of statutory principles that must apply to all actions and decisions taken on behalf of a person with incapacity. Dental professionals are required to apply these principles when providing care and treatment for a person who is incapable.

- A person must be assumed to have capacity unless it is established that they lack capacity.

   This principle upholds the autonomy of the person. It also means that as the presumption in law is that a person has capacity you do not need to assess the capacity of each patient you see. You are only required to assess capacity where there is a doubt in your mind about a patient's ability to make a decision.

- A person is not to be treated as unable to make a decision unless all practicable steps to help them to do so have been taken without success.

   The test for capacity requires a person to understand and use the treatment information given to them. This principle requires you to use simple practical steps to support the person such as a language the person understands, using pictures rather than words, waiting until the person is more alert, etc.

- A person is not to be treated as unable to make a decision merely because they make an unwise decision.

   The test for capacity requires that you are able to discern an impairment or disturbance to the person's mind or brain that might be affecting their decision-making ability. Where there is no impairment then you cannot take action under the Mental Capacity Act and must accept the decision as an unwise decision.

- An act done or decision made under this Act for or on behalf of a person who lacks capacity must be done, or made, in their best interests.

  Whenever a decision is made on or behalf of a person lacking capacity it must be made in that person's best interests. Where a dental professional believes that a decision maker is not acting in a person's best interests they may challenge that decision. If the conflict cannot be resolved then the Court of Protection can decide what is in the person's best interests.

- Before the act is done, or the decision is made, regard must be had to whether the purpose for which it is needed can be as effectively achieved in a way that is less restrictive of the person's rights and freedom of action.

  The Act, for the best of reasons, allows others to interfere in the lives of people who lack capacity. Human rights law allows such interference but only to the extent necessary to achieve a valid objective, such as health care. All actions under the Act must therefore be proportionate to the needs of the individual and all decisions must consider the rights and freedoms of the incapacitated person.

Decision-making capacity

Capacity to make decisions is the key to a person's autonomy and the Act sets out a test for decision-making capacity and the circumstances where a person would be regarded as incapable of making a decision.

The two-stage test

The Mental Capacity Act 2005 sets out a two-stage functional test based on the decision to be made at the time rather than a person's theoretical ability to make decisions generally. The dental professional will need to determine if there is:

(i) An impairment of or disturbance in the functioning of the person's mind or brain and, if there is,

(ii) The extent to which it affects the person's ability to make a decision by assessing whether the person is unable to:

  (a) Understand the information relevant to the decision or

  (b) Retain that information or

  (c) Use or weigh that information as part of the process of making the decision or

  (d) Communicate the decision (whether by talking, using sign language or any other means).

If the dental professional reasonably believes that the person fails any one or more of these four conditions then he or she can conclude that the person lacks capacity for this particular decision.

Designated decision makers

Where a dental professional reasonably believes their patient lacks capacity to decide on treatment then they must consider if a designated decision maker is in place who can consent on the patient's behalf.

The Mental Capacity Act 2205 allows a person to nominate another to make health and welfare decisions for them when they are incapable through a Health and Welfare Lasting Power of Attorney. Dental practices must keep a copy of the registered power of attorney document and ask the attorney for consent before proceeding with treatment in the same way they would ask a patient for consent.

On rare occasions where a person who lacks decision-making capacity has ongoing health and welfare needs, the court can appoint a deputy with power to consent to examination and treatment. Again the dental practice will need a copy of the deputy's authority to give consent, for the patient's records.

Treatment in an emergency

Patients are entitled to make consent to treatment decisions even when an emergency occurs. If the patient has capacity the dental professional must obtain consent before treatment can proceed. A patient can refuse consent even where a medical emergency arises and even where this will have serious consequences on the patient's health.

Where a patient lacks decision-making capacity such as when they are unconscious then the dental professional may act in their best interests out of necessity. Treatment may be given where it is immediately necessary to preserve life or prevent serious harm to the patient (*F v West Berkshire HA* [1990]).

Patients can however limit the treatment to be provided in an emergency through the use of advance decisions refusing treatment.

Advance decisions refusing treatment (ADRT)

This informal instrument can refuse dental treatment in advance. It can also be constructed to refuse life-sustaining treatment. For example if a patient had a valid and applicable ADRT refusing resuscitation in an emergency then the dental professional would have to respect the wishes of the patient if they were satisfied:

- That the ADRT was in writing;
- Was signed by the maker;

- Was witnessed in the presence of the maker;

- Contained a clear statement as to when it should apply; and

- Contained a statement from the maker stating that it was to apply even if their life was at risk.

Consent and children

Dental professionals will have children under 16 on their case load. In general the child will be seen with a parent or person with parental responsibility whose consent will be obtained before treatment (see Table 13.3).

The Children Act 1989, Section 2(9) allows a person with parental responsibility to arrange for someone else to exercise it on their behalf.

There is no requirement for this arrangement to be made in writing. For example, children may be brought for treatment by a person without parental responsibility such as a grandparent or childminder. In this situation, as long as the dental professional is satisfied that the person has the authority of someone with parental responsibility, then treatment can proceed with proxy consent.

Some children may seek treatment without their parents being present and dental professionals will need to decide if the child is able to give a valid consent to treatment.

Children reach the age of majority or adulthood at 18. However, while the courts acknowledge that no child under 18 is wholly autonomous, they do recognise the right of a child to consent to medical treatment as they develop and mature with age.

Age however is not the determining factor for decision-making capacity. In law, capacity is based on a person understanding and using treatment information. It is not based on a child reaching puberty.

The Gillick competent child

The issue over whether a child under 16 has the necessary capacity to consent to medical examination and treatment was decided by the House of Lords in *Gillick* v *West Norfolk and Wisbech AHA* [1986] and dental professionals must apply the rule in *Gillick* when determining whether a patient under 16 has capacity to consent to examination and treatment.

When determining whether a child has sufficient maturity and intelligence to make a decision the dental professional will need to take account of:

- the understanding and intelligence of the child;

- their chronological, emotional and mental age;

- their intellectual development; and

Table 13.3 Who has parental responsibility for a child?

Parental responsibility

Parental responsibility is defined as the rights duties, powers duties and responsibilities, which by law a parent has in relation to a child (Children Act 1989, s3)

Mother

Mother has automatic parental responsibility on the birth of the child (Children Act 1989, s2(1) and (2))

Father

Father has parental responsibility if he was married to the child's mother at the time of the birth (Children Act 1989, s2(1))
OR
If he subsequently married the mother of his child (Children Act 1989, s2(3); Family Law Reform Act 1987, s1) OR

If he became registered as the father of the child after 30 December 2003 (Children Act 1989, s4(1)(a)) OR

He and the child's mother make a parental responsibility agreement (Children Act 1989, s4(1)(b)) that is made and recorded in the form prescribed by the Lord Chancellor OR

The Court on his application orders that he shall have parental responsibility (Children Act 1989, s4(1)(c) OR

He obtains a residence order (Children Act 1989, s12 read with s4) OR

He is appointed as the child's guardian and the appointment takes effect (Children Act 1989, s5)

Acquired parental responsibility can only be removed by a Court

Others who can acquire parental responsibility

A person in possession of a residence order which could include the father of the child (Children Act 1989, s12)

A person appointed as the child's guardian once the appointment takes effect; this could include the father of the child (Children Act 1989, s5)

A person, other than a police officer, who is in possession of an emergency protection order (Children Act 1989, s44(4)(c))

A person who has adopted a child (Adoption Act 1976, s12 or Adoption & Children Act 2002, s46)

A Local Authority may additionally acquire parental responsibility

By obtaining a care order (Children Act 1989, s31)

By obtaining a freeing for adoption order (Adoption Act 1976, s18) or a placement order (Adoption & Children Act 2002, s21)

PROFESSIONAL AND LEGAL ISSUES

- their ability to reach a decision by appraising the advice about treatment in considering the nature, consequences and implications of that treatment (*Gillick* v *West Norfolk and Wisbech AHA* [1986] per Lord Scarman).

The aim of the rule in *Gillick* is to reflect the transition of a child to adulthood. Legal capacity to make decisions is conditional on the child's gradually acquiring the maturity and intelligence to be able to make treatment decisions. The degree of maturity and intelligence needed depends on the gravity of the decision. A relatively young child would have sufficient maturity and intelligence to be capable of consenting to a plaster on a small cut. Equally, a child who had the capacity to consent to dental treatment or the repair of broken bones may lack capacity to consent to more serious treatment (*Re R (A minor) (Wardship Consent to Treatment)* [1992]).

Decision-making capacity therefore does not simply arrive with puberty; it depends on the maturity and intelligence of the child and the seriousness of the treatment decision to be made.

A dental professional must be satisfied that a child has fully understood the nature and consequences of treatment before they can accept their consent or refusal of treatment. It is for the dental professional to decide whether or not a child is Gillick competent and able to consent to treatment. However, the power to decide must not be used as a licence to disregard the wishes of parents whenever the dental professional finds it convenient to do so. Those who behave in such a way would be failing to discharge their professional responsibilities and could expect to be disciplined by their professional body (*Gillick* v *West Norfolk and Wisbech AHA* [1986]).

Where a child is considered Gillick competent then the consent is as effective as that of an adult. This consent cannot be overruled by a parent.

Treating children in an emergency

The same doctrine of necessity applies when treating a child in an emergency as applied to adults under the same circumstances. The Children Act 1989 also allows the dental professional to do what is necessary in the interests of a child's welfare when having care of the child in an emergency (Children Act 1989, section 3(5)).

DUTY OF CONFIDENCE OWED TO PATIENTS BY DENTAL PROFESSIONALS

Whatever the age of the patient, dental professionals base their treatment on a thorough examination. This includes a personal history where details are disclosed on the basis that the personal information will be kept private and that the dental professional undertakes not to disclose it without permission.

The duty of confidence

There are three key areas that come together to reassure patients that the confidentiality of their health information will be respected.

1. A duty to respect patient confidentiality that is a specific requirement linked to disciplinary procedures in all NHS employment contracts and

underpinned by the NHS code of practice on confidentiality (Department of Health, 2003);

2. A legal duty that is derived from case law and supplemented by statute law (*Cornelius* v *DeTaranto* [2001]); and

3. A professional duty established by *Standards for Dental Professionals* (General Dental Council 2005a) and further supplemented by *Principles of Patient Confidentiality* (General Dental Council 2005b).

The duty of confidence is not, however, absolute. There will be occasions where confidential information about a patient will need to be disclosed to others. Such a disclosure must be to an appropriate person and comply with the requirements of the dental professional's contractual, professional and legal duty of confidence or they will be called to account and face sanction for breaching confidentiality.

It is essential therefore that dental professionals:

- understand the scope of the duty of confidence owed to the patients in their care; and

- disclose information even where given in confidence when it is right and proper to do so.

Contractual duty of confidence

All contracts of employment in the National Health Service must contain a clause imposing a duty of confidence on all staff that stresses that disciplinary action will result if that duty is breached (Department of Health, 2003). Similar clauses are included in the contracts of dental professionals working in private dental practices.

To discharge this duty dental professionals will need to show that:

- They will not disclose confidential patient information through inappropriate means such as gossiping;

- When they seek advice about a patient's treatment with a colleague they do so in private so that confidentiality is not inadvertently breached;

- They accurately record information received from and about their patients;

- They keep patient information and records private and physically secure;

- They only access information for the patients in their care; and

- They only disclose patient information to an appropriate source in accordance with the NHS code of practice on confidentiality, the requirements of the law and their code of professional conduct.

The duty extends to all patients, both past and present. Although there is no specific legal or professional requirement that states that a duty of confidence extends to deceased patients, the contractual duty extends confidentiality beyond the grave and includes those who have died.

The professional duty of confidence

The professional requirement for confidentiality is stipulated in the General Dental Council's *Standards for Dental Professionals* (General Dental Council 2005a).

Clause 3 states that dental professionals must guard against breaches of confidentiality by protecting information from improper disclosure at all times. This imposes a duty not to voluntarily disclose information gained in a professional capacity to a third party. This duty is enforced by the threat of professional discipline.

Confidence and the law

There is a legal obligation to respect patients' confidences that arises out of a general duty on everyone to keep confidential information secret.

A legal obligation of confidence arises when the information:

- Has the necessary quality of confidence; that is, the information is not generally available or known. Information of a personal or intimate nature qualifies (*Stephens* v *Avery* [1988]) and this is largely the type of information dental professionals receive from their patients.

- Has been imparted in circumstances giving rise to an obligation of confidence. In *Attorney General v Guardian Newspapers No 2* [1988] Lord Keith held that the law has long recognised that particular relationships gave rise to a duty of confidence. One of these was the dentist–patient relationship.

- Has been divulged to a third person without the permission and to the detriment of the person originally communicating the information. An invasion of personal privacy will suffice (*Duchess of Argyll* v *Duke of Argyll* [1967]). As it is in the public interest that medical confidences are kept secret the court will regard an unwarranted disclosure of patient information as detrimental (*Attorney General* v *Guardian Newspapers No 2* [1988]).

The duty of confidence is not absolute

Given the wide scope of the duty of confidence it is perhaps no surprise that dental professionals are reluctant to divulge information about their patients to others. Yet the contractual, professional and legal duties of confidentiality are not absolute and are subject to a range of exceptions that justify disclosure. It is important that dental professionals are aware of these exceptions in order to ensure that information is appropriately disclosed for effective care and protection of vulnerable patients while avoiding a charge of misconduct.

Consent of the patient

Permission to disclose confidential information from the person who originally imparted it is the starting point in law. The courts generally require this consent to disclosure to be in the form of an explicit consent preferably signed by the patient (*Cornelius* v *DeTaranto* [2001]). This ruling also reflects the requirements of the Data Protection Act 1998. The consent exception is only valid if the person knows exactly what information is to be disclosed and who is to receive the information.

Disclosure for treatment purposes

Confidentiality can be breached where information is shared with others concerned with the clinical care of the patient. Wide disclosure to any dental professional or doctor is not justified. To require an express consent from a patient each time their case was discussed would be impractical and even detrimental.

Where patients have consented to healthcare, research has consistently shown that they are content for information to be disclosed in order to provide that healthcare (National Health Service Information Authority, 2002).

Disclosing information when specifically asked to do so by a patient

When asked by a patient to pass on confidential information about them then the court regards this as a binding obligation. In *C* v *C* [1946] Justice Lewis considered the refusal of a sexually transmitted infection clinic to divulge information about a patient despite his request for disclosure. The judge held that, whilst it was important that proper secrecy be observed in sexually transmitted disease clinics, those considerations did not justify a health professional refusing to divulge confidential information to a named person when asked by the patient so to do.

Disclosing information without specific consent

The Department of Health advises that there are a number of exceptions allowing disclosure to appropriate sources without the consent of patient (Department of Health, 2003). These exceptions act as a useful aid when making a judgement about disclosing information concerning a patient.

Where a patient is incapable of receiving information or of consenting to disclosure, then disclosure of care and treatment information to the client's relative or main carer may be judged to be appropriate.

Disclosure to appropriate sources is allowed in cases of suspected abuse of vulnerable adults and children under vulnerable adult and child protection procedures. The public interest in protecting the welfare of children and the vulnerable will outweigh the duty to maintain a confidence (Department of Health 1999, 2002).

Disclosure in the public interest

The courts accept that when a case concerning disclosure of confidential information comes before them they are required to strike a balance between two competing interests: the public interest in keeping confidential information secret must be weighed against the public interest in allowing disclosure.

The public interest exception covers a broad range of situations including:

- Disclosure in the interests of justice;
- Disclosure for the public good;
- Disclosure to protect a third party; and
- Disclosure to prevent or detect a serious crime.

Disclosure in the interests of justice

A court has the power to order disclosure of confidential matters if it is in the interest of justice and refusing to do so would result in contempt of court. In *Attorney General* v *Mulholland* [1963] two journalists refused to name the sources of information in articles written by them. One of the journalists was sentenced to 6 months and the other to 3 months' imprisonment for contempt.

Dental practitioners, therefore, can be required by the courts to disclose information about their patients both in the form of written statements and in oral evidence where this is necessary in the interests of justice.

Disclosure for the public good

There may be circumstances where the public interest is served by disclosing information even though no crime has been committed or court action taken. This might include disclosing information to the proper authorities about a vulnerable adult or child.

Disclosure to protect a third party

Disclosure of confidential information may be necessary to protect a third party particularly where this concerns a vulnerable adult or child. The dental professional will need to consider the circumstances and use their professional judgement, informed by reference to the common law, to decide if the public interest in protecting the third party outweighs the public interest in keeping confidential information secret.

Disclosure to prevent or detect a serious crime

There may be circumstances when the dental professional is made aware that a patient is a victim of crime or has committed or intends to commit a crime. Before disclosing such information it will be necessary to weigh the seriousness of the crime against the countervailing public interest in maintaining patient confidentiality.

Disclosure is justified where the crime represents a real risk to public safety. That is, there must be a need to prevent or detect a serious crime to justify breaching patient confidentiality as the countervailing public interest in maintaining sensitive health information would generally outweigh disclosure (*W v Egdell* [1990]).

Data Protection Act 1998

The Data Protection Act 1998 applies to personal information held on computer or as part of a relevant filing system. This definition would include health records. Under the provisions of the Act a decision to disclose personal health information must be fair and lawful.

To be lawful the disclosure of personal health information must meet the requirements of the common law duty of confidence and be justified (Data Protection Act 1998, schedules 2 and 3).

Caldicott Guardians

Each NHS organisation has a guardian of person-based clinical information who oversees the arrangements for the use and sharing of clinical information. They ensure that patient-identifiable information is only shared for justified purposes and that only the minimum necessary information is shared in each case.

The Caldicott Guardian plays a key role in ensuring that the NHS satisfies the highest practical standards for handling patient-identifiable information. The Guardian will actively support work to facilitate and enable lawful and ethical information sharing.

PROFESSIONAL AND LEGAL ISSUES

Where a dental professional working in the NHS is unclear about whether a disclosure of information is justified they can seek advice from their Caldicott Guardian.

CONCLUSION

- Law and ethics are now fundamental to the practice of dentistry and underpin the dental practitioner's relationship with the profession and with his or her patients.

- A registered dental professional is legally and professionally accountable for their actions.

- Accountability to society is achieved through the public law that seeks to protect patients through the regulation of practice and the environment of care.

- General Dental Council (2005a) has acknowledged that medical emergencies can occur at any time so all members of staff must know their role in the event of a medical emergency.

- In an emergency certain prescription-only medicines may be supplied and administered without prescription.

- Dental professionals are also accountable to the individual patients in their care through the civil law.

- Dental professionals continue to owe their patient a duty of care in emergency situation and are expected to be able to respond effectively to the common emergencies that might arise in dental surgeries.

- Grossly negligent treatment which exposed a patient to the risk of death, and caused it, would constitute manslaughter.

- Where a patient dies in a dental surgery it will likely be an unnatural or sudden death and such deaths fall into the category that must be reported to the coroner.

- An employed dental professional is accountable to their employer through the contract of employment.

- The standards by which practitioners are judged and the General Dental Council considers the public are entitled to expect are set out in the *Standards for Dental Professionals*.

- A key requirement of the *Standards for Dental Professionals* concerns respect for patient dignity and choice.

- To be a valid defence to a claim of trespass, consent needs to be full, free and reasonably informed.

- Patients are entitled to make consent to treatment decisions even when an emergency occurs.

- Where a patient lacks decision-making capacity such as when they are unconscious, then the dental professional may act in their best interests out of necessity where treatment may be given if it is immediately necessary to preserve life or prevent serious harm to the patient.

- If a patient has a valid and applicable Advance Decision Refusing Treatment that refuses resuscitation in an emergency, then the dental professional would have to respect the wishes of the patient.

- The same doctrine of necessity applies when treating a child in an emergency as applied to adults under the same circumstances.

- There are three key areas that come together to reassure patients that the confidentiality of their health information will be respected in contract, the law and through the profession.

- The contractual, professional and legal duties of confidentiality are not absolute and are subject to a range of exceptions that justify disclosure.

- It is important that dental professionals are aware of these exceptions in order to ensure that information is appropriately disclosed for effective care and protection of vulnerable patients while avoiding a charge of misconduct.

REFERENCES

Airedale NHS Trust v Bland [1993] AC 789.
Appleton v Garrett [1997] 8 Med LR.
Attorney General v Guardian Newspapers No 2 [1988] 3 WLR 776 (HL).
Attorney General v Mulholland [1963] 2 QB 477.
Bayliss v Blagg & another (1954) 1 BMJ 709.
Bolam v Friern HMC [1957] 1 WLR 582.
Bolitho v City & Hackney HA [1997] 3 WLR 1151.
British Home Stores Ltd v Burchell [1980] ICR 303 (EAT).
C v C [1946] 1 All ER 562.
Chatterton v Gerson [1981] QB 432.
Ciarlariello v Schacter [1991] 2 Med. L. R. 391.
Cornelius v DeTaranto [2001] EWCA Civ 1511.
Council for the Regulation of Healthcare Professionals v General Dental Council [2005] EWHC 87.
Department of Health (1999) *Working together to safeguard children*. The Stationery Office, London.

Department of Health (2002) *No secrets: Guidance on developing and implementing multi-agency policies and procedures to protect vulnerable adults from abuse.* The Stationery Office, London.

Department of Health (2003) *Confidentiality: NHS Code of Practice.* Department of Health, London.

Donoghue v Stevenson [1932] AC 562.

Duchess of Argyll v Duke of Argyll [1967] Ch 302.

F v West Berkshire HA [1990] 2 A.C. 1 (HL).

Forman v Saroya [1992] EWHC 13.

General Dental Council (2005a) *Standards for dental professionals.* GDC, London.

General Dental Council (2005b) *Principles of patient confidentiality.* GDC, London.

Gillick v West Norfolk and Wisbech AHA [1986] AC 112 (HL).

Gold v Haringey HA [1998] QB 481.

Greenfield v Irwin (A Firm) [2001] EWCA Civ 113.

Harmer v Cornelius (1858) 5 CB 236.

Hope J. (1994) Fraud epidemic that costs NHS millions. *Daily Mail*; 1 December 1994: p. 26.

Kent v Griffiths [2001] QB 36 (CA).

Lewis FM, Batey MV (1982) Clarifying autonomy and accountability in nursing services. *Journal of Nursing Administration*; 12(9):13–18.

Maynard v West Midlands RHA [1984] 1 WLR 634 (HL).

National Health Service Information Authority (2002) *Share with care: Peoples views on consent and confidentiality of patient information.* NHSIA, London.

National Health Service Litigation Authority (2007) *Annual Report and Accounts 2007.* NHSLA, London.

Prendergast v Sam and Dee [1989] 1 Med LR 36.

Prescription Only Medicines (Human Use) Order 1997 (SI 1997/1830).

R v Misra & Srivasta [2004] EWCA Crim 2375.

R v Tabassum [2000] 2 Cr App R 328.

Re MB (Caesarean Section) [1997] 2 F.L.R. 426.

Re R (A minor) (Wardship Consent to Treatment) [1992] Fam 11.

Re T (Adult: Refusal of Treatment) [1992] 3 WLR.

Re U [2002] Lloyd's Rep Med 93.

Reynolds v North Tyneside Health Authority [2002] Lloyd's Rep Med 459.

Rideout RW (1983) *Principles of Labour Law*, 4th edn. Sweet & Maxwell, London.

Roe v Ministry of Health [1954] 2 QB 66 (CA).

Rouse v Squires [1973] 2 All ER 903.

Schloendroff v Society of New York Hospitals (1914) 211 NY 125.

Sidaway v Bethlem Royal Hospital [1985] AC 871.

Stephens v Avery [1988] Ch 449.

W v Egdell [1990] 2 WLR 471.

Williamson v East London & City HA [1998] Lloyd's Rep. Med.

Wilson v Swanson (1956) 5 DLR (2d) 113 (Canadian Supreme Court).

Yorkshire Evening Post (2008) Leeds dentist jailed for groping patient. *Yorkshire Evening Post*; 1 April 2008: p. 1.

PROFESSIONAL AND LEGAL ISSUES

Index